# The Healing Art of Connecting with Patients

Fahad Aziz

# The Healing Art of Connecting with Patients

Springer

Fahad Aziz
Madison, WI, USA

ISBN 978-3-032-03623-0 ISBN 978-3-032-03624-7 (eBook)
https://doi.org/10.1007/978-3-032-03624-7



This Springer imprint is published by the registered company Springer Nature Switzerland AG
The registered company address is: Gewerbestrasse 11, 6330 Cham, Switzerland

*To my father, Aziz—your strength and grace in adversity have always been my compass.*

*To my mother, Gul—your gentle kindness has instilled in me the true meaning of compassion.*

*To my wife, Misbah—your love is my guiding light, revealing the beauty and power of connection.*

*To my sons, Farhan and Ayaan—your innocence opens my eyes to wonder and teaches me anew each day.*

# Preface

In the quiet moments at the bedside, where words are scarce and emotions run deep, I have come to understand that medicine is more than science—it is relationship, presence, and grace. This book was born from those moments. It is a reflection of my journey as a physician and a fellow human being trying to make sense of suffering, healing, and the space in between.

Throughout my years in medicine—from early training in internal medicine to the emotionally demanding field of nephrology—I have witnessed the immense power of human connection. I have also seen how easily that connection can be lost amid the hum of machines, the press of time, and the weight of clinical protocol. Too often, we are trained to cure but forget how to care. We master the lab values and imaging findings but overlook the stories, fears, and hopes that define our patients as people.

This book is not a critique of medicine, but a call to its essence. It is a reminder that behind every chart is a story, behind every diagnosis is a life, and behind every patient is a human being longing to be seen.

I wrote this book for the medical students rushing from ward to ward, for the residents overwhelmed by decisions, for the attending physicians who feel distant from their original calling, and for every patient who has ever felt unseen. I wrote it to affirm what I believe with all my heart: that the human touch is not a luxury in medicine—it is its foundation.

Each chapter explores a facet of that touch—humility, mindfulness, compassion, communication, shared decision-making, and hope—what I have come to call "The Laws of the Human Touch." These are not abstract ideals but lived practices, taught to me by patients, mentors, and moments of failure and grace.

To heal is not only to alleviate disease—it is to connect, to witness, and to walk alongside another soul with reverence. That is the healing art this book seeks to reclaim.

Madison, WI, USA Fahad Aziz

# Acknowledgments

I'm truly thankful to Pam Lagomarsino for her kind and careful help with editing this book.

# Contents

# Introduction 1

The relationship between a medical provider and a patient is one of the most unique and vital connections we, as humans, have ever established. This bond is equally crucial for the patients and the medical providers who care for them. It is a relationship built on trust, empathy, and a shared goal of healing.

## The Erosion of the Human Connection in Modern Medicine

However, amidst the long years of rigorous training in medical schools and residency programs, we often overlook a critical component of this relationship—the "human touch." This oversight is not just a minor gap in medical training but a significant shortfall that can affect the core of patient care. By its nature, the medical profession is demanding. It requires an extensive understanding of complex biological systems, the ability to diagnose and treat various conditions, and the resilience to manage the emotional weight of life-and-death situations. Yet, in this intense focus on clinical and technical skills, the importance of empathy, compassion, and the ability to connect with patients on a human level is often diminished.

Dr. William Osler, widely recognized as a founding professor of Johns Hopkins Hospital and a pivotal figure in modern health care, underscored the significance of viewing the patient as an individual. He is famously quoted as saying, "It is much more important to know what sort of a patient has a disease than what sort of a disease a patient has" [10]. This profound insight suggests the success of medical treatment is not solely dependent on the correct diagnosis or the most advanced treatment plan, but also on understanding the patient's individual experiences, fears, and hopes.

Dr. Peabody, a celebrated physician, teacher, and clinical investigator, in his essay "The Care of the Patient," emphasized how hospital admissions often strip patients of their identity, reducing them to "that mitral stenosis in room two." This practical habit shifts focus from the person to the illness, risking the neglect of the patient's emotional and social complexities. For instance, Henry Jones, dealing with



F. Aziz, *The Healing Art of Connecting with Patients*,
https://doi.org/10.1007/978-3-032-03624-7_1

mitral stenosis, also lies awake worrying about his family. His anxiety, unaddressed, could hinder his recovery despite proper medications. A compassionate conversation and support may alleviate his worries more effectively than medications alone. While Henry's condition may intrigue medical staff, it's crucial to remember his humanity—his fears, hopes, and need for empathy. Emotional distress often impacts physical recovery, and small acts like easing a cough or providing encouragement can make a profound difference. True healing requires treating the person, not just the disease [11].

## A Personal Journey Through the Disconnect

The early days of medical school are often filled with excitement and the promise of mastering the art and science of healing. However, during this thrilling journey of discovery and growth, I received a subtle message: "Doctors and nurses should keep a professional distance from patients to prevent emotional and physical burnout." While this advice seemed wise and intended to protect those who devote their lives to caring for others, I soon realized it had a troubling undertone—a detachment that, if not addressed, could undermine the qualities that make a physician exceptional.

Empathy, compassion, and the ability to connect with patients are the essential foundations of medicine. However, this advice has led to a distancing from these vital human qualities, substituting them with a cold, almost mechanical method of patient care. While the goal was to protect oneself, the outcome has been concerning: a gradual and quiet erosion of the heart of medicine.

During my first year of medical school, I unexpectedly found myself on the other side of the hospital bed due to a severe case of malaria. I was admitted to the place where I was training to help others. What happened over the next few days taught me a lesson far deeper than any lecture or textbook could convey—about the significant difference between treating a disease and genuinely caring for a person.

The doctors and nurses caring for me were remarkable in their clinical skills. They meticulously noted every symptom and followed every protocol with care. I felt assured I was in good hands. However, as time passed, I sensed a disheartening absence—an emptiness that no medical expertise could fill. Patients, myself included, seemed to be treated as mere cases or clinical puzzles rather than as individuals with fears, hopes, and personal stories.

Lying in that emergency department bed, I couldn't shake the feeling of being just another entry in a medical chart, a problem to be solved rather than a person to be cared for. The empathy I desperately needed, the compassion that could have eased my worries, was missing. This clinical detachment, while ensuring the perfect execution of medical protocols, created a void in the healing process—one that could only be filled by what I realized was the most potent medicine of all: the "human touch."

This revelation hit me hard. Here I was, a future physician, witnessing the impact of a system that had lost sight of its essential purpose: to care for people. I saw myself not just as a patient but as a reflection of my potential future in medicine—a future where technical skills alone wouldn't suffice, and a lack of empathy could turn even the best care into something cold and impersonal.

This experience sparked my passion and determination to ensure the profession's demands never strip away my humanity. I understood true healing extends beyond the physical; it includes the emotional and psychological well-being of the patient. I realized a physician's role is not just to treat the body but to care for the whole person, providing medical expertise, comfort, reassurance, and a connection that goes beyond the clinical.

Navigating this disconnect was a pivotal moment in my understanding of what it means to be a physician. The experience shaped my perspective on medicine, highlighting that while the scientific aspects are crucial, the art of compassion and human connection truly bring the practice to life, elevating it from just a job to a meaningful vocation.

## The Importance of the Human Touch

The phrase "human touch" goes beyond just a physical gesture; it embodies the core values of empathy, compassion, and understanding that health care providers extend to their patients. It's the heartfelt act of holding a patient's hand, listening to their worries, or sharing comforting words during their most vulnerable times. While these gestures may seem small, they hold a significant, unspoken promise—that the patient is not alone in their journey and they are recognized, listened to, and cherished beyond their medical conditions.

Dr. Rachel Naomi Remen, a renowned physician and author, beautifully expresses this idea: "The practice of medicine is not about curing diseases; it is about caring for people." This viewpoint encourages us to rethink the conventional approach to medicine, which frequently emphasizes just the diagnosis and treatment. It invites health care professionals to move past clinical detachment and adopt a more comprehensive perspective on healing—one that considers patients' emotional and psychological well-being alongside their physical health.

Imagine a patient resting in a clean hospital room, surrounded by the sounds of machines and the busy rhythm of medical staff. They are not just patients in bed; they face fear, uncertainty, and perhaps a deep loneliness. In these moments, a gentle human touch can serve as a lifeline, providing hope in an otherwise sterile environment. The presence of a medical provider willing to connect on a personal level can turn this experience from isolation into one of meaningful connections.

This gap between the technical side of health care and the emotional needs of patients raises an important question about the essence of healing: Is it sufficient to simply treat the illness, or should we also consider the patient's deeper emotional and psychological needs? Research consistently indicates that patients who feel understood and cared for by their doctors are more likely to follow treatment plans, experience less anxiety, and report greater satisfaction with their care [8, 14, 15]. These insights highlight the significant impact a human touch can have on a patient's journey through illness.

Without a human touch, even top-notch medical care can be cold and distant. It helps patients feel appreciated, boosts their spirits, eases their pain, and restores their dignity. The human touch transforms treating an illness into genuinely healing a person. While technology and innovation are important, they can't replace the unique and timeless bond formed with patients. It truly is the heart of medicine, nurturing trust, care, and healing.

## The Consequences of Neglecting the Human Touch

Neglecting the human element in medicine isn't just a small mistake; it's a significant issue that can profoundly affect patients and health care providers in troubling ways. For patients, a lack of empathy and compassion can lead to feelings of isolation, where fear and mistrust can take hold. Picture a patient who is already feeling vulnerable and scared, stepping into a health care environment that views them merely as a collection of symptoms or a problem to fix. When a medical provider focuses only on the medical record instead of the individual in front of them, it fosters a feeling of invisibility—an unsettling sense they are not genuinely seen or listened to.

This sense of disconnection can have serious effects. When patients feel misunderstood or unappreciated, they might hold back important details about their symptoms or worries, fearing they won't be taken seriously or thinking it won't make a difference. This can result in misdiagnoses, delays in treatment, and ultimately, less-than-ideal outcomes. Moreover, the lack of a caring connection can worsen feelings of anxiety, depression, and hopelessness, especially for those facing a long-standing diagnosis of a chronic disease or life-threatening illnesses. These patients are not only fighting their conditions but also dealing with the emotional burden of feeling isolated in their journey, feeling let down by the very system meant to support them.

For health care providers, ignoring the importance of human connection can also lead to serious issues, though they show up differently. Medical provider burnout is becoming a widespread problem in the medical field, a quiet crisis that affects the well-being of those who commit themselves to healing others. At its heart, burnout is often tied to the emotional strain of caring for patients day after day without building meaningful relationships. When the human touch is missing, medicine can turn into a mechanical, draining process—a never-ending cycle of diagnosis and treatment that lacks personal fulfillment.

## The Mastery of Sir Joseph Bell: A Lesson in Observation and Humanity

Sir Arthur Conan Doyle, famous for creating the beloved detective Sherlock Holmes, found inspiration in an extraordinary real-life figure: Sir Joseph Bell. Bell, a Scottish surgeon and lecturer at the University of Edinburgh, was anything but an ordinary doctor. His exceptional talent for combining sharp observation with genuine empathy made him a legend among his students. For those lucky enough to learn from him, Bell was not just a skilled diagnostician but also a remarkable teacher who grasped the true essence of healing beyond mere science. One particular story highlights the depth of his methods and the lasting impact they had.

On a typical day in the outpatient department, patients waited their turn while Bell sat with eager medical students. Among the arrivals was a woman with her child, appearing quite ordinary at first. She greeted Bell with a simple "Good morning." But what happened next left everyone in the room in awe.

Without any introductions or background, Bell asked, "What sort of crossing did you have on the ferry from Burntisland?"

The woman, taken aback, replied, "It was good."

Bell continued seamlessly, "And what did you do with the other child?"

Her surprise grew. "I left him with my sister at Leith," she answered.

Then he asked, "Did you take the shortcut down Inverleith Row to get here to the infirmary?"

"Yes, I did," she confirmed, now completely bewildered.

"And are you still working at the linoleum factory?" Bell inquired.

"I am," she said, her astonishment increasing.

As his students watched in amazement, Bell turned to them to explain the method behind what seemed like magic. "When she said, 'Good morning,' I immediately recognized her Fife accent," he noted. "The nearest ferry crossing from Fife is from Burntisland, so I inferred she took that ferry. The coat she carries is too small for the child with her, indicating she started her journey with two children but left one behind. The red clay on her shoes is unique to the area near the botanical gardens, which she must have passed by, taking the shortcut down Inverleith Row. Lastly, the dermatitis on her right hand is common among linoleum factory workers in Burntisland."

The students were in awe. In just moments, Bell had constructed a detailed narrative about the woman's life, journey, and work—all without any medical instruments or extensive questioning. He showcased the power of observation and the importance of truly seeing the patient as a person rather than just a collection of symptoms.

Bell's demonstration was more than just a display of his observational prowess; it was a profound lesson in the art of medicine. He illustrated that healing goes beyond treating physical ailments. By understanding a patient's context—where they come from, what they do, and their challenges—medical providers can build deeper connections with those they serve. For Bell, observation was not just a diagnostic tool but a means to bridge the gap between medical provider and patient, fostering trust and empathy.

For Sir Arthur Conan Doyle, this moment became a key element of Sherlock Holmes's character, whose legendary deductions were inspired by Bell's real-life brilliance. For Bell's students, it was a vivid reminder of what it means to practice medicine: to look beyond illness and see the individual.

This timeless story of Sir Joseph Bell is even more relevant in today's technology-driven health care landscape. Modern medicine has made incredible advancements, with sophisticated diagnostics, robotic surgeries, and AI tools becoming commonplace. However, as Dr. Abraham Verghese, an American physician and author, pointed out in his TED talk "A Doctor's Touch," these innovations can sometimes overshadow the most vital aspect of healing: human connection. Verghese emphasized, "The most important innovation in medicine to come in the next 10 years: the power of the human hand, the human touch, the human connection."

Bell's approach highlights that true healing involves not only addressing physical illnesses but also considering the emotional and social needs of patients. His knack for understanding a patient's story through careful observation reminds him that no technology can replace the medical provider's role as a compassionate listener and observer.

At its heart, Bell's legacy is a powerful testament to the significance of empathy in medicine. His ability to see beyond clinical details and connect with patients as human beings reminds us that medicine is both a science and an art. His story teaches us that the human touch is not just an accessory to care but essential for health care providers and patients. It uplifts spirits, fosters trust, and restores dignity, ensuring that healing remains profoundly human [6, 8, 12, 16].

## Reclaiming the Human Touch in Medical Practice

Reclaiming the human touch in medical practice doesn't mean we have to give up the scientific principles that support modern medicine. Instead, it's about understanding science and compassion go hand in hand—they complement each other beautifully. The true essence of medicine is found in our ability to blend these two aspects: using scientific knowledge while showing empathy and caring for the whole person rather than just focusing on the illness.

As I advance in my medical career, I am increasingly convinced that the human touch is a crucial part of the healing process. It enables us to connect with our patients, to truly hear their fears and concerns, and to offer care that is not only effective but also filled with compassion. The challenge for everyone involved in health care—educators, practitioners, and students alike—is ensuring this important element of care isn't overlooked in the fast-paced world of modern medical training and practice. By doing so, we can create a health care environment where patients and medical providers can flourish and where the art of healing is approached with expertise and heartfelt care.

## Defining the Human Touch

The "human touch" in health care is about more than just medical expertise; it transforms clinical interactions into meaningful experiences. It's about genuinely understanding a person's pain and walking alongside them on their journey. This connection bridges the gap between clinicians and patients, promoting empathy and compassion instead of distance.

This approach goes beyond simply understanding a patient's condition—it involves a sincere desire to share their fears, acknowledge their vulnerabilities, and see them as individuals rather than just their illness. While building this type of connection can be emotionally demanding for medical providers, it's a courageous choice that enriches the patient's experience and the physician's sense of purpose.

During the tumultuous Crimean War (1853–1856), where injured soldiers filled overcrowded and unsanitary hospitals, disease and despair often claimed more lives than battle injuries. In this grim reality, one remarkable figure emerged as a symbol of hope and compassion: Florence Nightingale. Her story is not just about medical reform; it highlights the incredible power of human connection—a legacy that still inspires medicine today. The situation was dire when Nightingale arrived at the British military hospital in Scutari in 1854. Soldiers lay on bare floors, suffering in agony amidst filth and vermin. The air was thick with decay, and infectious diseases like cholera and typhus were rampant, leading to a staggering 42% death rate among the injured. Morale was at an all-time low.

For many, this scene seemed hopeless—a battlefield where the wounded were left to die in silence. But for Florence Nightingale, it was a call to action. With determination, courage, and a belief in the value of every human life, she set out to transform not only the conditions but also the very spirit of the place. Nightingale and her team of nurses worked tirelessly to enhance the hospitals. She implemented groundbreaking changes: cleaning the wards, improving ventilation, and ensuring basic sanitation. She advocated for fresh food and clean water—luxuries in such a grim environment. However, her unwavering dedication to the soldiers' emotional well-being truly made her efforts impactful. When the day's chaos subsided at night, Nightingale would stroll through the dimly lit wards, lamp in hand. She would stop at each bed, speaking gently to the soldiers, providing comfort and reassurance. Her presence became a source of solace, her compassion a balm for their suffering. Soldiers referred to her as "The Lady with the Lamp," who brought light to their surroundings and spirits.

Nightingale's efforts had a significant impact. Within 6 months, the hospital's death rate plummeted from 42% to just 2%. Her careful record-keeping and data-driven approach to reform established the groundwork for modern public health practices. Yet her true legacy extended beyond statistics; it was about restoring dignity and humanity to those reduced to mere war casualties. For the soldiers, Nightingale was more than a nurse; she was a beacon of hope. Her gentle touch and kind words assured them they were not forgotten and someone cared about their suffering. She listened to their fears, wrote letters for them to their families, and sat with those who were dying, ensuring no one faced their final moments alone. Her human touch transformed a place of despair into one of healing.

Florence Nightingale's story is a powerful reminder that medicine and caregiving are as much about compassion as they are about knowledge. Her kindness, despite overwhelming adversity, illustrated that the human touch could illuminate even the darkest situations. It emphasized that healing involves addressing the emotional, psychological, and spiritual needs of the person behind the symptoms.

Nightingale's legacy continues to resonate in modern medicine, where technology often risks overshadowing human connection. The human touch, exemplified by Nightingale's relentless efforts, is not merely an addition to care—it is the core foundation of true healing. It lifts spirits, restores dignity, and reaffirms the profound bond between caregiver and patient. Nightingale's lamp still shines brightly, guiding all who strive to infuse humanity into their work in medicine [4, 5, 7, 9].

## The Impact of "Human Touch" on Physician Burnout

As a nephrologist, I have often encountered the profound impact of human suffering in medicine. I work with patients dealing with kidney failure, a complex condition that carries both health risks and emotional burdens. Managing this illness demands medical expertise and a reservoir of empathy, patience, and emotional resilience. Many of these individuals rely on hemodialysis, a crucial treatment that teeters on the fine line between life and death.

During my nephrology fellowship at the University of Missouri, I encountered the stark reality of this illness. The alarming mortality rates among hemodialysis patients were not just statistics; they represented real lives lost, families affected, and dreams shattered. What impacted me even more was the overwhelming sense of hopelessness that pervaded the dialysis unit, creating an atmosphere heavy with despair and a silent acknowledgment of the relentless nature of this disease.

In the midst of this suffering, I also observed a troubling detachment among my health care colleagues. Doctors and nurses, once full of passion for their work, appeared to be weighed down by their responsibilities. Their conversations shifted from lively discussions about saving lives to somber talks about exhaustion and burnout. They spoke of their desire to escape, planning vacations as if a brief getaway could mend their emotional strains.

Listening to these exchanges, I couldn't help but wonder: Is stepping away from the workplace truly the answer to burnout? Can a short retreat heal the deep wounds caused by constant exposure to suffering and loss? I feared the answer was no.

Burnout in medicine is not just a result of being overworked; it reflects a deeper disconnection from the very purpose that drives many of us to this field: the wish to heal and make a difference in the lives of those in need. When that connection fades and medicine becomes a mechanical task devoid of human touch, burnout often follows.

But what if the solution to burnout is not escaping our work but changing how we engage with it? What if, instead of distancing ourselves from our patients' suffering, we embraced it, connecting with them on a profoundly human level? Could this human connection—truly sharing our patients' experiences—be the remedy for the emotional fatigue that often burdens health care providers?

Research indicates it might be. Studies have shown that medical providers who believe in the human touch—who see their patients as individuals with unique stories, fears, and aspirations—experience lower levels of burnout. This meaningful connection can provide a powerful source of fulfillment, reminding us of the significant impact we can have on others' lives [1].

For me, this realization was both enlightening and humbling. I began to understand that caring for my patients and genuinely connecting with them was more than just a duty—a source of emotional nourishment. In those moments of authentic connection, when I could look into a patient's eyes and offer more than medical guidance, I rediscovered my sense of purpose. During these interactions, the weight of burnout lifted, replaced by a fulfillment that no vacation could ever match.

The positive effect of the human touch on medical provider burnout is not merely a theory; it is a lived experience. It highlights that while health care can be demanding, it can also be incredibly rewarding when approached with empathy and compassion. By embracing the human aspect of care and engaging with our patients personally, we can enhance patient outcomes and shield ourselves from the emotional toll that often leads to burnout.

Ultimately, it is not about escaping our responsibilities but connecting—finding meaning in the work that challenges us. The human touch serves as a remedy not just for our patients but for ourselves, helping to keep the flame of purpose alive even in the most challenging times.

## A Lesson from My Mentors: The Power of Connection

In the wide world of medical education and practice, some enlightening moments can change the trajectory of our careers and lives. One such significant moment came from a remarkable man whose wisdom and genuine compassion matched his unwavering commitment to his patients—Dr Ramesh Khanna, the nephrology chairman at the University of Missouri. He wasn't just a mentor but a shining example of what it means to be truly connected to those we care for.

Dr. Khanna was a remarkable man who dedicated decades to medicine, navigating the many challenges that came his way. He encountered countless patients, each with unique stories and struggles, and through it all, he fostered a deep connection with everyone he met. What truly distinguished him was his medical knowledge and perspective of seeing patients as individuals deserving of kindness, respect, and love.

He consistently showed me that building meaningful relationships with patients was not merely a nice gesture but the heart of being a healer. In those connections, Dr. Khanna discovered the real significance of his work. He illustrated that the intricate science of nephrology could only be fully appreciated when approached with an open heart. He taught me that medicine goes beyond prolonging life or alleviating pain; it's about being present in the lives of those we care for, sharing in their joys and sorrows, and providing more than just medical care—offering hope.

I observed Dr. Khanna interacting with his patients not just as a physician but as a friend, a confidant, and sometimes even a surrogate family member. He remembered their names, stories, fears, and dreams. He knew when to speak and when to listen. His office was adorned with thank-you notes, photos, and tokens of appreciation from patients whose lives he impacted, not just through his medical skills but through his genuine humanity.

As the years went by, I recognized these connections were not only beneficial for his patients; they were what nourished him. Dr. Khanna retired at the impressive age of over 80 after a fulfilling career that couldn't be measured by awards or titles, but rather by the love and kindness exchanged. His approach was a living example that the secret to a long and rewarding medical career lies not in avoiding the stresses of the profession but in fully embracing them—by cultivating deeper, more meaningful relationships with patients.

For me, Dr. Khanna's message was unmistakable: the true essence of medicine is found not in the tools or techniques we employ but in the human connections we forge. These connections transform a job into a calling, prevent burnout, and turn a career into a cherished journey.

Upon starting my training in transplant medicine at the University of Wisconsin, I was filled with enthusiasm, determination, and a heartfelt aspiration to heal illnesses and deeply care for individuals. Little did I know then that my journey would be greatly influenced by a remarkable person—Dr Arjang Djamali.

Dr. Djamali wasn't just an expert in transplant nephrology, but a master of connection. From the beginning, I noticed something different about how he engaged with his patients. He didn't just review their charts or adjust their medications—he sat with them and asked about their lives, families, and fears. He knew their stories: where they came from, what they loved, what kept them up at night. For Dr. Djamali, each patient was a person first and a clinical case second.

I recall entering a clinic room one morning with him. The patient, a woman in her 50s who had recently faced allograft failure, seemed visibly worried. Dr. Djamali didn't rush with questions or give cold instructions; instead, he greeted her warmly and with genuine interest. He inquired about her daughter's wedding plans, her church choir, and her favorite recipes. Her expression changed—she seemed more at ease, as if she had briefly escaped the weight of her illness and found solace in being truly understood. This wasn't an act; it was simply who he was. He paid attention to details, listened attentively, and made time for people even when the clinic was busy or the consult list was long. I observed families drawn to him not only for his expertise but also for the sense of comfort he brought to the room.

And then there were times of sorrow—those unavoidable, deeply upsetting moments when, despite all efforts, the treatments were unsuccessful. Kidneys stopped functioning. Lives ended. What resonated with me the most was this: families cherished his kindness even while facing death. They didn't just express gratitude for his medical efforts—they appreciated his demeanor toward their loved ones. The empathy, support, and consistent respect he showed them during the most challenging times made an impact that no result could diminish.

In Dr. Djamali, I saw the kind of doctor I aspired to be. Not one is defined only by their clinical acumen, but by their capacity to make space for sorrow, joy, and connection. He taught me that our legacy in medicine is not written only in patient outcomes, but in the humanity we bring to the people we serve.

As I continue my career path, I carry the invaluable lesson Dr. Khanna and Dr. Djamali shared—a reminder that the core of medicine is not located in textbooks or labs but in the shared human experience between medical providers and their patients. In these moments of connection, we discover not only the strength to heal others but also the strength to heal ourselves.

## Personal Reflections on the Importance of Compassion

Life's journey often takes us through different roles in health care—sometimes we are caregivers, and other times, we seek care. In those vulnerable moments, whether for ourselves or our loved ones, we truly experience the incredible impact of the human touch in medicine, a force that's unforgettable.

In 2011, my father faced an unexpected challenge—triple vessel bypass surgery. The weight of the situation was heavy on our hearts, casting a shadow of fear and uncertainty over our family. As a physician, I understood the risks and complexities of such a major surgery. Yet, as a son, I felt a different fear—of being powerless in the presence of something so significant.

During the agonizing hours before the surgery, it wasn't the technical details that comforted us. It was the human element of the surgeon and the nursing staff—their reassuring words, calm voices, and warm presence. With his steady hand and kind eyes, the surgeon spoke to our hearts as much as our minds. "We will take care of him," he said, and his conviction eased some fear I felt. The attentive and gentle nursing staff offered their skills and their humanity, providing a comforting presence that brought more relief than any medication could.

In those moments, I truly grasped the transformative power of the human touch. It wasn't just about alleviating my father's pain or ensuring a successful surgery; it was about soothing the emotional turmoil that accompanies such experiences. It was about giving us the strength to hope when hope felt fragile. This compassion didn't just comfort us—it fortified us, helping us face the uncertainty ahead.

Then, in 2018, the situation reversed. My younger son, my precious child, experienced a febrile seizure. The terror of that moment is something no parent should endure—the sight of your child convulsing, the fear gripping you, the helplessness weighing you down. As we rushed to the emergency department, my mind raced with worst-case scenarios, my heart pounding with dread.

But amidst the chaos, a calm presence emerged in the form of an emergency doctor. His kind words, delivered with authority and understanding, were like a soothing balm to my frantic heart. "Your son is in the right place," he said, reassuringly touching my shoulder. "We will take care of him." Those simple yet profound words washed over me like a wave of peace. At that moment, I knew my son was in capable hands—not just medically, but emotionally. The human side the doctor showed was more than professional courtesy; it was a lifeline that pulled me back from the depths of fear.

These experiences have profoundly shaped my perspective. I've learned that while patients and their families may not always remember the names or faces of their caregivers, they will never forget the human touch and comfort they received. Human touch in medicine isn't a luxury; it's a necessity. It transforms a frightening clinical environment into a sanctuary of hope and healing.

In the grand tapestry of medicine, the human touch is the thread that ties everything together. It gives meaning to the science, breathes life into the practice, and ultimately defines the experience for both patient and caregiver. My experiences have convinced me that, in the end, it's not the technical skills or academic achievements that leave the deepest impact—it's the human touch, kindness, and compassion that resonate in the hearts of those we serve.

## The Debate: Is Medicine an Art or a Science?

The ongoing discussion about whether medicine is an art or a science has been around for as long as the field, engaging scholars, practitioners, and patients. Some believe medicine is fundamentally a science rooted in empirical evidence, thorough research, and systematic problem-solving. Others argue it's an art requiring intuition, creativity, and a profound understanding of human experiences. In reality, medicine encompasses both aspects, and it's in the harmonious blend of these two that the essence of healing emerges.

On the one hand, the scientific foundation of medicine underpins all medical practices. Science equips us with the knowledge to diagnose illnesses, comprehend their underlying causes, and create life-saving treatments. The remarkable advancements in medical technology, pharmacology, and surgical methods showcase science's ability to enhance human health. It is precise and logical, often revealing the intricate complexities of the human body, serving as the cornerstone of modern health care, and empowering physicians to address even the most demanding medical challenges.

However, science alone, despite its precision and strength, falls short. The art of medicine—the human element—infuses life into this science, transforming clinical interactions into meaningful healing experiences. This artistic side enables medical providers to look beyond mere symptoms, recognizing patients as whole individuals with distinct fears, hopes, and emotions. It's this artistry that fosters deep connections with patients, providing comfort during difficult times and instilling hope even amidst uncertainty.

The art of medicine transcends good bedside manner; it embodies intuition, empathy, and the skill to navigate the intricacies of human emotions. It acknowledges that each patient is not just a case to be solved, but also a life deserving of care. This aspect requires a unique skill set—one that textbooks and labs can't teach. It calls for physicians to engage their humanity, listen with their hearts, and be fully present with their patients.

Dr. Albert Schweitzer is a remarkable example of how the art and science of medicine can unite to change lives. Born in 1875 in Germany, Schweitzer was already a celebrated theologian, philosopher, and musician when he made the bold decision to pursue medicine at 30. Despite his accomplishments in other fields, he felt a deep moral calling to dedicate his life to alleviating suffering in underserved communities.

In 1913, Schweitzer and his wife, Helene, relocated to Lambaréné, Gabon, which was then part of French Equatorial Africa, where they encountered significant health challenges, such as malaria and dysentery, with minimal access to medical care. He set up a makeshift hospital along the Ogooué River, starting with a rundown chicken coop as a treatment area. With limited resources, Schweitzer often had to think quickly, using whatever was available to provide care. His scientific background enabled him to treat diseases and perform surgeries under tough conditions, while his compassion and determination earned the trust of the local community.

Schweitzer's approach was deeply influenced by his philosophy of "Reverence for Life," which held that all living beings deserve respect and care. This principle guided every aspect of his work, shaping his scientific efforts and relationships with patients. He treated everyone with dignity, viewing his work as a service to humanity. His hospital became a refuge for the sick, offering not only medical treatment but also emotional and spiritual support. Schweitzer often took the time to converse with patients, listen to their stories, and address their fears. For him, healing was more than curing illness; it was about restoring hope and dignity. Schweitzer faced numerous challenges in Lambaréné, including being interned as an enemy alien during World War I due to his German nationality.

Nevertheless, he remained resolute, returning to Lambaréné post-war to rebuild and expand the hospital with global donor support. Over the years, his hospital evolved from humble beginnings into a well-respected medical center, serving thousands annually. His relentless dedication earned him the Nobel Peace Prize in 1952, recognizing his extraordinary contributions to humanity.

Schweitzer's life exemplifies the powerful impact of blending scientific knowledge with a deep "human touch." He demonstrated that medicine is not just a technical field but a deeply human one. His work in Lambaréné reminds us that healing involves more than tools and expertise; it requires a genuine connection with people, understanding their challenges, and offering hope. Through his philosophy of reverence for life, Schweitzer illustrated that medicine is both an art and a science, with human connection at its core. His legacy continues to inspire health care professionals to look beyond physical ailments and address the emotional and spiritual needs of their patients [2, 3, 13].

The discourse around art and science in medicine is not one that needs resolution, but rather one that needs to be embraced. It's in the interplay of these two forces that the true power of medicine is realized. The human touch transforms the cold logic of science into something warm, compassionate, and profoundly effective, making health care not just a profession but a calling.

Ultimately, medicine is about more than just curing diseases; it's about caring for people. It combines the science that helps us understand with the art that enables us to heal. And it's in this delicate balance that the true magic of medicine resides.

## Framing the Journey: The Structure of This Book

In the complex and high-stakes field of medicine, where choices can significantly impact a person's life, certain doctors excel beyond just technical expertise. They are more than body specialists; they are caretakers of the spirit. These exceptional medical professionals possess a unique talent: the skill to form deep connections with their patients on a personal level. They recognize that while medical knowledge is crucial, it is not complete without the art of caring. Their effectiveness is not only in their medical expertise or accuracy of diagnosis but in their ability to provide solace in times of uncertainty, support in moments of fear, and empathy even when solutions seem elusive. These instances often shape a career—and, at times, a life.

Throughout my journey, I have been fortunate to witness the quiet excellence of such individuals. What left an enduring impact was not only their skill but also their humanity: the gentle hand on a shoulder, the unhurried conversation at the bedside, and the ability to hold space for sorrow without rushing to fix it. These were not random acts of kindness. They were guided by principles—deliberate, embodied actions rooted in a more profound philosophy of care.

Over time, I recognized these patterns and named them "The Laws of the Human Touch." These laws are not abstract ideals. They are intentional practices that shape how we show up for others in moments of vulnerability. They are the habits of heart and mind that distinguish good physicians from great healers. They protect us from burnout, deepen our impact, and remind us of the sacredness of our work.

This book is structured around these core principles. It is divided into *three interconnected parts*, each representing a phase in the evolution of a healer—from inward reflection to outward connection to ultimate transformation. Together, these parts form a roadmap for reclaiming the humanity of medicine—for ourselves and for those we serve.

## Part 1: The Inner Landscape of a Healer

Before we touch others, we must first understand ourselves.

This part begins where all healing must begin—from within. In a profession that often prizes detachment as a form of self-preservation, these chapters ask us to turn inward—with humility, presence, and vulnerability. They challenge us to examine how we present ourselves to patients—not just our knowledge, but also our intentions and emotional availability.

Here, we explore two foundational laws: humility and mindfulness.

- **Humility** teaches us that we are never above learning—from our patients, our mistakes, and the human condition itself.
- **Mindfulness** invites us to slow down and be fully present—to listen not only with our ears but with our attention and intention.

Without these qualities, even the most skilled clinician can become detached or mechanical. But with them, we build a grounded presence—a steady emotional center from which all healing flows.

## Part 2: Building Human Connections

Healing flows through connection—when words, tone, and presence align with intention.

Once we are grounded in self-awareness, we can extend outward. This part explores how to translate inner clarity into meaningful relationships with those we care for. Healing, after all, is not a solitary endeavor—it emerges in the space between two people.

This part examines three essential laws: *compassion, communication*, and *shared decision-making*.

- **Compassion** moves us to recognize suffering and act to relieve it—not out of obligation but from a place of deep empathy.
- **Communication** is more than relaying information; it is the bridge that turns understanding into trust.
- **Shared Decision-Making** honors the autonomy of our patients, transforming care into a partnership rooted in respect.

These chapters are practical, relatable, and emotionally resonant. They show how small, intentional moments—an attentive pause, a validating response, a collaborative plan—can turn clinical encounters into transformative connections.

## Part 3: Transforming Through Hope

To offer hope is to remind someone that the future is still theirs.

The final part of this book focuses on what may be the most elusive yet powerful force in healing: *hope*. This part contains a single law but combines all the previous ones in an emotionally resonant culmination.

Hope is not about denying reality. It is about offering light within it. It is the quiet courage to sit beside someone in their darkest hour and whisper, with presence more than words: "You are not alone."

Hope can look like honesty, tenderness, or perseverance. It can be the difference between giving up and holding on. And remarkably, it doesn't just heal patients—it revives us, too.

This chapter explores how hope becomes the sustaining force—for patients navigating the uncertain path of illness and for physicians striving to find meaning in suffering. It reminds us that we can still care even when we cannot cure. Even when we cannot change the outcome, we can still change the experience.

This book is more than a reflection on best practices. It is an invitation—to slow down, be present, and lead with your humanity. It is a call to rediscover what drew us to the field in the first place: the desire not just to fix but to serve.

As you read, I encourage you to reflect on your journey. When did someone's compassion reshape your path? When did a patient, mentor, or family member remind you that healing is as much about connection as it is about cure?

Together, let us walk through these laws—not simply to become more competent clinicians but to become more whole, present, and human.

## Conclusion

In a world where medicine increasingly leans on technology, algorithms, and efficiency, the quiet power of the human touch remains its most transformative force. This chapter has traced a journey—through personal stories, historical legacies, and scientific evidence—to illuminate a truth we must not forget: Healing is not merely a technical endeavor but a human one.

To treat without compassion is to care for a body, not a person. Yet when we look into a patient's eyes and genuinely see them—not as a diagnosis, but as a fellow human in need—we restore dignity to our work and their experience. Medical professionals like Osler, Peabody, Bell, Nightingale, Schweitzer, and modern-day mentors remind us that the greatest medicine we possess is not in prescriptions but in presence, empathy, and genuine connection.

This chapter calls us to remember why we chose this path: not just to cure but also to care. As we move forward in our work, may we carry this conviction with us: the human touch is not an accessory to healing—it is its foundation.

**Take-Home Points**

- Empathy and compassion are as crucial as medical expertise in patient care.
- Treat patients as individuals, not just diagnoses or symptoms.
- Human connection prevents burnout and restores purpose for health care providers.
- Holistic healing integrates physical, emotional, and psychological care.
- Reclaiming compassionate care is essential for meaningful medical practice.

## References

1. Aziz F. Compassionate care essential for better clinical outcomes, burnout prevention. WMJ. 2023;122(3):160–1. https://www.ncbi.nlm.nih.gov/pubmed/37494641
2. Brabazon J. Albert Schweitzer: a biography. 2nd ed. Syracuse: Syracuse University Press; 2000.
3. Cicovacki P. The restoration of Albert Schweitzer's ethical vision. London: Continuum International Pub; 2012.
4. Cook E. The life of Florence Nightingale. London: Macmillan; 2012.

5. Dossey BM. Florence Nightingale: a 19th-century mystic. J Holist Nurs. 2010;28(1):10–35. https://doi.org/10.1177/0898010109356474.
6. Edwards W. The real life Sherlock Holmes: a biography of Joseph Bell – the true inspiration of Sherlock Holmes and the Pioneer of forensic science. Scotts Valley: CreateSpace Independent Publishing Platform; 2013.
7. Fee E, Garofalo ME. Florence Nightingale and the Crimean War. Am J Public Health. 2010;100(9):1591. https://doi.org/10.2105/AJPH.2009.188607.
8. Hojat M, Louis DZ, Markham FW, Wender R, Rabinowitz C, Gonnella JS. Physicians' empathy and clinical outcomes for diabetic patients. Acad Med. 2011;86(3):359–64. https://doi.org/10.1097/ACM.0b013e3182086fe1.
9. Nightingale F. Notes on nursing: what it is, and what it is not. London: Harrison and Sons; 1859.
10. Osler W. Aequanimitas, with other addresses to medical students, nurses and practitioners of medicine. Philadelphia: P. Blakiston's Son & Co., Inc.; 1932.
11. Peabody F. The Care of the Patient. JAMA. 1927;88:877–82.
12. Raffensperger J. Was the real Sherlock Holmes a pediatric surgeon? J Pediatr Surg. 2010;45(7):1567–70. https://doi.org/10.1016/j.jpedsurg.2010.03.006.
13. Schweitzer A. Out of my life and thought: an autobiography. Baltimore: Johns Hopkins University Press; 2009.
14. Stewart MA. Effective physician-patient communication and health outcomes: a review. CMAJ. 1995;152(9):1423–33. https://www.ncbi.nlm.nih.gov/pubmed/7728691
15. Street RL Jr, Makoul G, Arora NK, Epstein RM. How does communication heal? Pathways linking clinician-patient communication to health outcomes. Patient Educ Couns. 2009;74(3):295–301. https://doi.org/10.1016/j.pec.2008.11.015.
16. Verghese A. A doctor's touch. 2011. https://www.ted.com/talks/abraham_verghese_a_doctor_s_touch/transcript?subtitle=en

# Part I

# The Inner Landscape of a Healer

*Before we touch others, we must first understand ourselves.*



*This section grounds the reader in the inward qualities needed to be fully present and open to others—an emotional and mental preparation for the healing journey.*

# 2 Humility

Dr. Meera Patel moved swiftly through the hallways of the university hospital, her white coat fluttering behind her like a cape. As a dual-trained infectious disease and internal medicine physician, she was often called the "Sherlock Holmes" of the consult service. She'd developed a reputation for finding answers where others had reached dead ends.

On Tuesday morning, she got a page from the oncology floor about a 68-year-old woman named Joan Michaels, who had been experiencing fevers for over a week. They had started her on broad-spectrum antibiotics as a precaution. However, the blood, urine, and sputum cultures returned negative. A CT scan also excluded pneumonia, abscess, and any serious abdominal issues. The team was puzzled, but Dr. Patel found the case fascinating.

She reviewed the medical record quickly on her iPad outside the room: recent diagnosis of stage II breast cancer, completed chemotherapy 3 months ago, now admitted with intermittent fevers, fatigue, and malaise, and workup thus far was unrevealing.

Classic fever of unknown origin, she thought.

As she entered the room, she found Mrs. Michaels sitting upright in bed, her frame slight and her face pale but composed. A scarf covered her hair, which had not fully grown back. Her medical record said "cachectic," but Dr. Patel saw something else—an alertness, a spark.

"Good morning, Mrs. Michaels. I'm Dr. Patel from Infectious Diseases. I've come to help figure out what's causing your fevers," she said, her tone brisk but warm.

Joan smiled faintly and nodded. Then she did something unusual. She reached out and gently placed her hand on Dr. Patel's.

"Doctor," she said quietly, "may I tell you my story before we begin?"

Dr. Patel hesitated. She had four more consults to see before noon. Her pager buzzed. But there was something in how Joan said it—something human, urgent,


F. Aziz, *The Healing Art of Connecting with Patients*,
https://doi.org/10.1007/978-3-032-03624-7_2

and unquantifiable. Dr. Patel slid the clipboard onto the windowsill and pulled up a chair.

"Of course," she said.

Joan began slowly. "Six months ago, I lost my husband. He was my world. He was a Vietnam veteran, and he'd been sick for years. He had this strange disease no one could name—something with granulomas, I think. After he died, I started feeling off. My energy dropped. I got these odd rashes, and I forgot things. I thought it was grief. Then the cancer diagnosis came, and everything else got pushed aside."

Dr. Patel listened, scribbling nothing, interrupting nothing.

"I know the tests haven't shown much," Joan continued. "But I feel like there's something deeper going on. Something we're not seeing."

When the story ended, Dr. Patel sat in silence for a moment. Then she began a new line of questioning—more personal, more contextual. She asked about travel, exposures, and any history of autoimmune disease. Something about the mention of granulomas and systemic symptoms triggered a quiet suspicion.

Back in the workroom, she requested a battery of labs—ESR, ANA, ANCA, ACE levels, and serum calcium. She ordered a high-resolution CT and a tissue biopsy of a peculiar skin lesion Joan had mentioned in passing. Her resident raised an eyebrow.

"You think it's sarcoidosis?"

"I don't know yet," Dr. Patel replied, "but her story suggests we're missing something."

Two days later, the pathology confirmed cutaneous sarcoidosis. Joan's fevers were inflammatory, not infectious. The antibiotics were stopped. Steroids were initiated. Within 72 h, her fevers disappeared, her appetite improved, and she smiled for the first time during rounds.

Later that week, at a departmental conference, a colleague praised Dr. Patel for "thinking outside the box."

But she gently corrected him.

"It wasn't me," she said. "She gave me the diagnosis. I just finally sat down and listened."

Dr. Patel's journey isn't focused on rare diseases or exceptional diagnostic skills. It's about humility—the kind that allows a health care provider to put their ego aside, take a moment, and truly listen to what the patient knows but hasn't had the chance to share.

As we delve into history, we discover that during the early nineteenth century, medicine was evolving rapidly, and many diagnostic tools we rely on today were yet to be invented. A notable advancement was made by a young French doctor, Dr. René Laennec, who saw the difficulties in his practice and was motivated to discover a more effective way to care for his patients.

Dr. Laennec served at the Necker-Enfants Malades Hospital in Paris, a prominent institution of his era. He was a skilled physician with a deep knowledge of pathology, but he recognized the limitations of the diagnostic tools of his time. Back then, doctors mainly relied on percussion and auscultation to listen to heart and lung sounds, but these methods had drawbacks. Percussion, which involved tapping on the chest, often missed underlying issues, while auscultation—listening directly to the chest—could be quite challenging, especially with larger patients or those whose conditions made it difficult to hear the delicate heartbeats and lung sounds.

One day, Dr. Laennec encountered a patient who would significantly impact the future of medicine. A young woman was admitted with symptoms of a heart condition, and it was essential to make an accurate diagnosis. As was his usual practice, Laennec attempted to listen to her heart by placing his ear on her chest. However, her weight made it difficult for him to hear the sounds.

Rather than succumbing to frustration or settling for the limitations of this approach, Laennec took a moment to think things through. He recognized that directly placing his ear on her chest wasn't the most effective way to detect heart sounds, especially when layers of tissue posed a challenge. Inspired by a wave of creativity and innovation, Laennec sought a better solution, not just relying on his abilities but also considering a simple external tool that could elevate his diagnostic efforts.

As Laennec reflected on his challenge, he recalled an observation from his earlier days. While caring for patients in his youth, he used a rolled-up piece of paper to enhance sounds when trying to listen to something from afar. This sparked a simple yet brilliant idea: why not apply a similar method to hear heartbeats better? He quickly crafted a tube from the rolled-up paper and placed it on the patient's chest. Through this tube, the sounds of the heart were amplified, allowing Laennec to hear much more clearly than before.

This humble innovation, though simple in design, marked the birth of the stethoscope—a significant instrument in the history of medicine. By adopting a common, everyday object to serve a vital medical purpose, Laennec demonstrated the power of humility and creativity in medical practice. Instead of relying solely on existing methods or his ego, he embraced the idea that there might be a better, more efficient way to serve his patients.

Laennec's discovery soon gained popularity in the medical community. With his humble attitude, he shared a comprehensive overview of his invention in his 1816 publication, *De l'Auscultation Médiate* (On Mediate Auscultation). In this work, he explained how to use the stethoscope and emphasized its importance in diagnosing heart and lung diseases. The stethoscope allowed doctors to listen more effectively, especially for internal conditions like pleurisy, pneumonia, and tuberculosis—diseases that were often difficult to detect.

While many viewed Laennec as a pioneer in diagnostic medicine, he stayed remarkably humble regarding his role in developing the stethoscope. In his writings, he didn't seek personal accolades; instead, he emphasized the significance of listening to patients and the importance of keen observation. He recognized the stethoscope was not a means to elevate his medical status, but rather a tool to improve patient care by attuning to their internal voices.

Dr. René Laennec's journey is more than just creating a legendary medical tool; it's a testament to humility when faced with obstacles. Laennec illustrated that the heart of medical practice is in our readiness to reflect, innovate, and truly listen—not only to the body's sounds but also to our patients' voices. With his invention,

Laennec showed us that the most effective solutions often come from recognizing our limitations and working to enhance the lives of others [5, 6, 8].

## Defining Humility in Health Care

Humility is an essential quality for anyone in the health care profession. It shapes how medical providers connect with patients, collaborate with colleagues, and deliver care. At its core, humility involves recognizing no one possesses all the answers and there's always room for growth and learning. In health care, this translates to being open to the perspectives and experiences of others, including patients, fellow doctors, and new research findings.

- **Humility vs. Self-deprecation:** While humility involves acknowledging our limitations, *self-deprecation* goes further by sometimes downplaying our abilities or worth. In the health care field, genuine humility enables a medical provider to admit when they are unsure or need assistance while still appreciating their expertise and confidence in their role. Conversely, self-deprecation can foster doubt, potentially affecting patient care or decision-making.
- **Intellectual Humility—Acknowledging What We Don't Know:** A medical provider who adopts an approach of humility isn't hesitant to admit when unsure about a diagnosis or treatment plan. They actively seek advice, listen to their colleagues, and stay updated on medical advancements. This eagerness to learn from others enables medical providers to deliver better care and continuously improve their practice.
- **Cultural Humility—Respecting Patients' Lived Experiences:** Cultural humility is about embracing each patient's unique experiences, backgrounds, and values. It acknowledges that a person's health beliefs and actions are influenced by their culture, family, and personal history. By practicing cultural humility, medical providers take the time to appreciate a patient's perspective and honor their values, even when these differ from their own.
- **Interpersonal Humility—Viewing the Patient as a Partner:** Interpersonal humility involves viewing patients as individuals who follow instructions and as partners in their treatment. This approach emphasizes treating patients respectfully, actively listening to their concerns, and including them in health-related decisions. It creates a relationship where patients feel acknowledged, appreciated, and empowered to participate actively in their care.

## The Dangers of Ego in Medicine

In medicine, having confidence in one's skills is important, but it's also crucial to keep ego and arrogance in check. While being knowledgeable and self-assured helps provide excellent patient care, an overblown sense of self-importance can hinder essential elements of good health care, such as empathy, collaboration, and patient safety. When health care professionals let their ego guide their choices, they might overlook the patient's experience and the valuable insights of their colleagues, which can lead to less favorable outcomes. Arrogance can often result in dismissive attitudes and a failure to listen, ultimately undermining the trust and respect vital for effective health care.

Empathy is vital in creating strong relationships between medical providers and patients, but an arrogant attitude can hinder that connection. When medical providers focus solely on their expertise, they may overlook their patients' emotional and psychological needs, which can lead to a lack of meaningful engagement. This affects the quality of care and can leave patients feeling unheard and misunderstood. As a result, failing to build an empathetic relationship can lead to poorer patient experiences and lower contentment with care.

In the health care setting, teamwork is key; yet a medical professional's ego can pose a significant challenge to this collaboration. Medicine thrives on effective communication and mutual respect among all team members, including nurses, specialists, and support staff. When a provider's ego overshadows the importance of teamwork, it can lead to dismissive attitudes toward others' input, breaking down trust within the health care team, creating a less efficient environment, and potentially making it unsafe for patients. Effective teamwork, built on equal collaboration and respect, is essential for providing the best care.

Finally, patient safety is paramount, and arrogance can jeopardize it. Medical errors often happen when providers ignore their limitations or hesitate to seek help due to their ego. Such behavior can lead to overlooking critical signs or failing to verify important decisions, ultimately putting patient health at risk. When a health care professional's ego stands in the way of collaboration or seeking second opinions, it can result in treatment delays, misdiagnoses, and even life-threatening situations. In medicine, prioritizing patient well-being over ego is essential for a safer and more effective health care system.

A powerful historical lesson in the importance of humility in medicine comes from the life and work of Dr. Ignaz Semmelweis, often called "the savior of mothers." In the 1840s, Semmelweis was working at the Vienna General Hospital, where two maternity wards existed side by side—one staffed by doctors and medical students and the other by midwives. He noticed something deeply troubling: Women giving birth in the doctors' ward were dying at significantly higher rates from puerperal fever (childbed fever) than those in the midwives' ward.

Semmelweis investigated the differences between the two clinics and made a groundbreaking observation: Doctors and students frequently went directly from performing autopsies to delivering babies without washing their hands. He hypothesized they were carrying cadaverous particles from dead bodies to living mothers. Though germ theory had not yet been developed, Semmelweis instinctively instituted a handwashing policy using chlorinated lime solution. The results were astonishing—mortality rates in his clinic dropped from over 10% to below 2%.

But instead of being hailed for his discovery, Semmelweis faced intense backlash from the medical community. His peers refused to accept that their own unclean hands could cause death. Acknowledging this required humility, and many were unwilling to embrace it. Physicians—esteemed, educated, and respected—were not ready to consider they might be harming patients. His findings were rejected, ridiculed, and labeled unscientific. Eventually, he was dismissed from his position, and his ideas were largely ignored until years later, when Louis Pasteur's germ theory and Joseph Lister's antiseptic techniques validated his conclusions. Tragically, Semmelweis died in an asylum, having spent his final years fighting against the arrogance that silenced the truth.

This story is not just about one man's insight; it is about the institutional failure to practice humility. It is a cautionary tale that exposes the fatal cost of arrogance in medicine. Had Semmelweis's colleagues responded with curiosity instead of contempt—had they admitted they didn't have all the answers—thousands of lives might have been saved much earlier [4, 7].

The story highlights an essential truth: *humility in medicine is a sign of wisdom, not weakness*. It acknowledges that no single doctor has all the solutions, and advancement comes from being open to listening, asking questions, and accepting the possibility of being wrong. Back in Semmelweis's era, lives were lost due to a refusal to acknowledge an uncomfortable truth. Today, we still face that risk whenever pride overshadows curiosity, and teamwork and seeking second opinions are viewed as a challenge instead of a helpful resource.

In April 2019, Chad Gerlaugh, a quadriplegic man from Tampa, Florida, went in for what was thought to be a routine kidney stone surgery at Morton Plant Hospital. Unfortunately, the procedure took an unexpected and tragic turn. After the surgery, Gerlaugh developed sepsis, which can lead to organ failure and even death if not treated swiftly.

Despite showing signs of infection, the medical team did not respond as quickly or effectively as needed. It wasn't until Gerlaugh's condition deteriorated significantly that the seriousness of his infection was acknowledged, but by that time, significant harm had already occurred. The delay in treatment resulted in multiple amputations—both legs above the knee and one arm above the elbow. In 2021, Gerlaugh filed a medical malpractice lawsuit against the hospital and its doctors, alleging they failed to recognize the seriousness of his sepsis and respond appropriately.

This case brought attention to a lapse in medical judgment and the potential risks associated with overconfidence. The physician involved may have been too self-assured in handling a complex situation, neglecting the importance of thorough reevaluation and seeking second opinions. This oversight in recognizing their limitations and acting promptly resulted in irreversible consequences. The lawsuit emphasizes the critical need for humility and swift action when faced with medical challenges and the necessity for a health care system that places patient safety above individual confidence [20].

In a heartbreaking story, 13-year-old Martha Mills from the UK was hospitalized in 2021 following a cycling accident. Initially, her injury appeared to be standard, but as her symptoms worsened, her parents grew increasingly worried and raised concerns. Unfortunately, their worries were not taken seriously by the medical staff. As Martha's health declined, the critical signs of sepsis went unrecognized by the doctors.

By the time Martha's condition was accurately evaluated, it was too late; the delay in diagnosing her sepsis resulted in organ failure, and she tragically died. This incident sparked important discussions about the need for humility in health care. The medical team's inability to fully consider the family's concerns and conduct further investigations stemmed from a lack of openness. If the doctors had been more attentive and set aside their assumptions, they might have identified the sepsis sooner and possibly saved Martha's life.

Martha's untimely passing led to the creation of "Martha's Rule" in the UK, a law designed to empower patients and their families to seek a second opinion if their concerns are being overlooked. This initiative aims to prevent similar tragedies by ensuring health care professionals actively listen to patients and their families. It represents a commitment to fostering humility in health care through better communication and collaborative decision-making [9].

These cases are important reminders of how arrogance in medicine can lead to serious issues, highlighting humility's vital role in avoiding medical errors. In these situations, overconfidence resulted in a failure to listen to patients and their families and a hesitance to seek assistance or second opinions when challenges arose. In both Gerlaugh's and Mills' cases, the medical professionals involved either overestimated their diagnoses or overlooked others' concerns, which ultimately caused significant harm to patients.

By promoting a culture of humility and collaboration, health care professionals can help minimize the chances of these incidents occurring. A system that values listening to patients, acknowledging their concerns, and seeking further input when needed will ultimately enhance patient care and lead to safer outcomes.

## Humility and the Therapeutic Relationships

Humility is essential in the relationship between health care providers and patients. It goes beyond just medical knowledge and creates an atmosphere where patients feel appreciated, listened to, and actively involved in their care. When health care professionals show humility, they acknowledge their limitations and understand they don't have all the answers. This openness fosters a collaborative relationship, enabling the patient and provider to work together for better health results. Humility builds trust and strengthens their connection, leading to a deeper bond.

In health care, there's often a traditional power dynamic where the provider holds authority while the patient is more passive. However, humility helps to balance this dynamic. Humble providers view patients as partners rather than mere subjects, acknowledging patients are experts in their own lives and can offer valuable input about their care. By respecting and valuing a patient's autonomy, providers empower them to take an active role in their treatment decisions, creating a more collaborative and balanced relationship.

Dr. Virginia Apgar, an American obstetrical anesthetist, is celebrated for creating the Apgar score, a straightforward yet transformative tool for swiftly evaluating the health of newborns. Before her innovation, there were limited standardized methods for assessing neonates right after birth. Many distressed infants either weren't evaluated quickly enough or, when assessed, missed the timely interventions that could save their lives. Introduced in 1952, Dr. Apgar's score system significantly improved neonatal care by enabling quick decisions about whether a newborn required immediate medical attention.

What truly sets Dr. Apgar apart is not just the brilliance of her score but also the humility she displayed in her research and clinical practices. She didn't rely solely on her medical training but actively engaged with various health care professionals. By collaborating with nurses, pediatricians, and other specialists who worked closely with newborns, she listened to their insights and suggestions. Dr. Apgar understood that no one person has all the answers, and she appreciated the value of shared knowledge and teamwork in finding better solutions.

Her dedication to developing the Apgar score was fundamentally about enhancing patient care. Dr. Apgar prioritized improving outcomes for newborns over seeking personal accolades. Despite the worldwide impact of her score, she never pursued fame or recognition. Her main goal was to ensure babies, especially those born in distress, received timely and accurate evaluations to inform immediate care. This patient-focused mindset enabled her to emphasize the well-being of infants and equip health care professionals with the necessary tools for swift and effective decision-making during critical moments.

The significance of the Apgar score is immense. It has saved countless lives over the years and is utilized globally, every minute of every day, to assess newborn health. It is a fundamental component of neonatal care in hospitals worldwide, and its simplicity and effectiveness have made it a widely adopted diagnostic tool. Through her humility, Dr. Apgar established a scientifically robust system rooted in the practical experiences of those directly caring for newborns. Her story exemplifies how humility in health care—being receptive to others' contributions and prioritizing patient care over personal recognition—can lead to remarkable advancements in medical practice and improved patient outcomes [1, 10].

One of the most powerful and deeply personal examples of humility reshaping the therapeutic relationship comes from Dr. Rana Awdish, a critical care physician at Henry Ford Hospital in Detroit. In 2016, her life changed in an instant. Seven months pregnant, she was rushed to the hospital with a catastrophic hemorrhage caused by a ruptured liver tumor. She lost her unborn baby, suffered multi-organ failure, underwent multiple surgeries, and spent time on life support in the very ICU where she usually worked.

But what stayed with her most—long after the tubes were removed and her body recovered—was not just the trauma of the illness but the emotional and spiritual wound created by how she was treated as a patient.

Even as a physician, Dr. Awdish experienced her pain being downplayed, her inquiries overlooked, and her sense of self fading away in the health care system. It appeared clinicians prioritized laboratory results and clinical guidelines over recognizing the genuine fear, grief, and confusion she was going through. "We spoke the same language," she shared in interviews, "but I felt invisible." She remembered instances when the physicians' certainty and clinical detachment created a barrier—not only to comfort but also to the healing process itself.

This experience shattered her assumptions about what good care looked like. Before her illness, she admits, she believed in the ideal of the "flawless physician"—the expert who always knew the answer, maintained emotional distance, and controlled the conversation. But as a patient, she learned what she needed most wasn't answers—to be seen, heard, and held with compassion.

That required humility. In her memoir *In Shock*, she writes, "The real healing began the moment someone sat beside me, acknowledged the unknown, and just listened without trying to fix it."

Dr. Awdish now speaks nationwide, urging health care providers to abandon the performance of perfection and embrace a more human model of care—one grounded in humility. She argues humility is not a weakness but a pathway to genuine connection because it allows clinicians to approach each patient with curiosity, openness, and respect. It will enable patients to share what matters most to them—not just what is biologically wrong, but also what is emotionally or spiritually at stake.

Her story reveals therapeutic relationships are not built solely through knowledge or clinical skill but through presence, empathy, and the courage to be human. She said, "I thought I became a better doctor by knowing more. But I became a healer the moment I realized I didn't have to know everything. I just had to care."

Through the lens of her suffering, Dr. Awdish uncovered a more profound truth: Humility is the bridge that allows providers to cross from clinical expertise to compassionate *connection*. And in that space—where patient and doctor meet not as expert and subject, but as two humans facing uncertainty together—true healing begins [2, 3].

## The Humble Medical Provider: Traits and Practices

Humility in health care is more than just showing kindness or patience; it encompasses embracing certain qualities and actions that foster trust, collaboration, and growth within a clinical setting. A humble health care provider recognizes their limitations, is open to learning from others, and prioritizes the well-being of their patients above all else. Here are the traits and practices that characterize a humble clinician:

- **Active Listening Without Interrupting**

A humble medical provider listens to patients, colleagues, and staff without cutting them off. This involves giving full attention to the speaker, allowing them to express their concerns, thoughts, and feelings freely, without judgment or immediate replies. Active listening shows respect for the speaker's viewpoint and helps build trust. By dedicating time to listen attentively, clinicians can better understand their patients' needs, enabling them to make well-informed decisions. It also creates a space where everyone's voice is acknowledged and appreciated, resulting in more teamwork in care and greater patient satisfaction.

In 2018, Dr. Abraham Verghese, a renowned physician and author, shared a powerful story during a TED talk that perfectly illustrates the importance of active listening in health care and how humility plays a crucial role. Dr. Verghese, who specializes in internal medicine, has long advocated for a return to patient-centered care, focusing on diagnosing the disease and genuinely listening to the patient.

During his talk, Dr. Verghese shared an experience with a patient who had been suffering from an undiagnosed illness for months. The patient had visited multiple doctors, but no one could determine the cause of his symptoms. As a new physician, Dr. Verghese decided to step back and simply listen to the patient's narrative. He didn't interrupt, didn't try to solve the problem immediately, and instead allowed the patient to speak at length about their concerns.

As the patient spoke, Dr. Verghese's humility and active listening uncovered a crucial detail that the patient had not shared before—a subtle but significant symptom that the previous doctors had missed. This key piece of the puzzle led Dr. Verghese to the correct diagnosis. By simply listening, without rushing or interrupting, Dr. Verghese identified the illness and established a deeper rapport with the patient, which fostered trust and improved the therapeutic relationship.

This story demonstrates the profound impact of active listening in health care. Dr. Verghese's humility in allowing the patient to share their experience without judgment or interruption helped him uncover a diagnosis that had eluded others. His example highlights how essential it is for health care providers to listen actively and humbly, enabling them to provide more effective care while strengthening the doctor-patient relationship [22].

- **Admitting Errors and Sharing Decision-Making**

Humility in medicine means being open about mistakes and involving patients in decision-making. A humble medical provider embraces their errors, viewing them as valuable learning and improvement opportunities. This openness fosters trust and demonstrates integrity. It also promotes teamwork by encouraging a collaborative environment where everyone can share their knowledge. Additionally, when medical providers engage patients in discussions about all available options, risks, and benefits, it empowers them to take an active part in their care.

A wonderful illustration of humility in the medical field comes from the efforts of Dr. Atul Gawande, a well-respected surgeon, author, and public health authority. In his book *The Checklist Manifesto* (2009), Dr. Gawande highlights the significance of teamwork, acknowledging mistakes, and collaborative decision-making in health care. He points out that even with the extensive knowledge of health care providers, the world of medicine is rife with complexities and uncertainties, making errors a natural part of the process.

A striking instance of Dr. Gawande's approach to humility came during his involvement in a project to improve patient safety in surgery. Gawande's team implemented a simple yet effective checklist in hospitals worldwide to prevent errors during surgery. The checklist covered basic but often overlooked aspects, such as confirming the patient's identity and ensuring the surgical team communicated clearly about the procedure. Using checklists allowed health care providers to admit that no matter how experienced they were, they could not do everything perfectly and needed a system to prevent mistakes.

One particular story Dr. Gawande shares in his book is about a patient who was scheduled for elective surgery, and the team, despite being highly experienced, missed a crucial detail about the patient's previous medical history. The error was identified at the last moment due to a team member's willingness to speak up and the structured use of the checklist. Dr. Gawande candidly admitted that without the checklist, the team would have missed this critical information, leading to potential harm to the patient. This incident exemplified how acknowledging the possibility of mistakes and using systems to prevent them could save lives, even in the most routine procedures.

Dr. Gawande's humility in openly discussing the role of mistakes in surgery and his commitment to involving patients and their families in discussions about their care has impacted how medicine is practiced. His approach underscores the value of humility in admitting errors and emphasizes the importance of shared decision-making, empowering patients to play an active role in their care [12].

Dr. Brian Goldman, an experienced emergency physician and medical journalist from Toronto, has dedicated many years to one of the most intense areas of health care: the emergency department. Throughout his career, he has built a reputation as a skilled and calm clinician. However, what truly distinguishes Dr. Goldman is his willingness to openly discuss something many doctors tend to keep under wraps: his medical mistakes.

In his well-known TED talk, "Doctors Make Mistakes. Can We Talk About That?" (2011), Goldman shares a heartfelt story from the early days of his career. He was treating a middle-aged woman who came in with shortness of breath. Even though the signs pointed to congestive heart failure, he convinced himself she was just experiencing an asthma attack. She was sent home with a bronchodilator, but sadly, she died hours later due to the misdiagnosis.

Instead of suppressing the memory or blaming the system, Dr. Goldman reflected on his choices and what led to the mistake. He realized that part of the issue stemmed from the medical culture, which values certainty, shuns vulnerability, and discourages open discussions about errors. In this setting, many doctors feel alone, embarrassed to acknowledge their mistakes, and reluctant to share their uncertainties with others.

"Every doctor makes mistakes," he noted. "But not every doctor talks about them. And if we don't talk about them, how do we ever learn from them?"

His experiences ignited a vital discussion in the medical field. He has since become a national advocate for open error disclosure, supporting changes in institutions that encourage health care providers to own up to mistakes, learn from them, and engage patients in discussions about what went wrong and the next steps.

Goldman also highlights how humility is essential for shared decision-making. When a physician is open to saying, "I don't have all the answers," it invites the patient into the conversation. This fosters a dynamic where patients feel empowered to ask questions, voice concerns, and take an active role in their care. It creates equality, transforming the physician from an all-knowing authority into a trusted ally.

In his interviews and books like *The Night Shift* and *The Power of Kindness*, Goldman reflects on how his perspective on medicine has evolved. He now routinely asks patients what worries them, what they understand about their condition, and how they want to move forward. That simple act of listening—honoring the patient's voice—has made him a better doctor and a more compassionate person [11, 13–15, 23].

- **Welcoming Feedback from Peers, Staff, and Patients**

A caring medical provider is always eager to receive feedback from a range of sources, such as colleagues, staff, and patients. This willingness to listen is essential for personal development and enhancing the quality of care. Being humble here means recognizing no one has all the solutions, and input from others can provide valuable perspectives on improving. By embracing constructive criticism, health care professionals can sharpen their skills and adjust their practices to better serve their patients' changing needs. Moreover, inviting patient feedback creates a respectful and open environment, demonstrating that their thoughts and experiences are valued.

A recent and powerful example of humility, feedback, and shared decision-making in health care can be found in the work of Dr. Mona Hanna-Attisha during the Flint Water Crisis in Michigan. In 2014, a public health crisis unfolded when the drinking water in Flint was contaminated with lead, exposing thousands of children to the dangers of lead poisoning. Dr. Hanna-Attisha, a pediatrician and public health advocate, became a key figure in exposing the crisis and ensuring the affected communities received the care they needed.

Dr. Hanna-Attisha was initially met with skepticism from local and state authorities when she raised concerns about the high lead levels in the water. Instead of allowing this resistance to silence her, she actively listened to the affected families, taking their concerns seriously and using their feedback to shape her advocacy. She worked tirelessly to gather data, seeking input from other professionals, including scientists, health care providers, and community leaders, to better understand the full extent of the crisis. Her humility in recognizing the limits of her expertise and her willingness to welcome feedback from a broad range of sources were crucial in driving change. By involving the community in discussions and listening to their stories, she could address their needs better.

In a pivotal press conference where she revealed her findings, Dr. Hanna-Attisha humbly acknowledged the uncertainty surrounding some data, but felt it was essential to speak out because of the urgency of the situation. She welcomed expert and community feedback, adapting her approach based on their input. This openness fostered trust within the community, and her commitment to transparency and collaboration made her an effective advocate for the residents of Flint. She also demonstrated the importance of involving the community in the decision-making process, ensuring the affected families were part of the solution and had a voice in their health care decisions.

Dr. Hanna-Attisha's approach to welcoming feedback and engaging in shared decision-making exemplifies humility and the power of collaboration in health care. Her actions helped uncover a public health disaster and ensured the community's voices were heard, valued, and integrated into addressing the crisis. Her ability to accept feedback from all stakeholders and remain flexible in her approach significantly impacted her, showing that humility, transparency, and patient-centered care are essential to effective health care advocacy [16].

Another example from the early 2000s would be Dr. Peter Pronovost, a critical care physician at Johns Hopkins, who discovered a concerning issue in American hospitals: central line-associated bloodstream infections (CLABSIs). These infections, which were often due to preventable errors during catheter placement, were causing numerous patient deaths and incurring significant health care costs. Despite clear guidelines, adherence was not uniform, and the medical community appeared resigned to these infections as an unfortunate aspect of hospital care.

Pronovost refused to settle for the current situation. Instead of assigning blame or giving orders from the top, he showed humility and curiosity. He reached out to frontline workers like nurses, residents, and bedside staff and posed a straightforward yet groundbreaking question: "What obstacles are hindering us from getting this right consistently?"

What he heard was concerning. Nurses had observed instances where doctors did not follow sterile procedures, such as not washing their hands or taking shortcuts during catheter insertions. However, they often felt unable to address these issues due to the established medical hierarchies. On the other hand, doctors were often pressed for time and sometimes didn't realize the impact of these seemingly minor shortcuts. Pronovost realized the existing system did not prioritize safety; it was based on tradition and authority rather than feedback and teamwork. Instead of ignoring this feedback or implementing strict measures, Pronovost collaborated with his ICU team to create a straightforward five-step checklist for central line insertion:

1. Wash hands with soap.
2. Clean the patient's skin with chlorhexidine.
3. Use sterile drapes.
4. Wear a sterile gown, gloves, mask, and cap.
5. Avoid using the femoral vein unless necessary.

Importantly, nurses were given the authority to stop the procedure if any step was skipped—a radical move when nurses were rarely empowered to challenge physicians.

This wasn't just about following a list—it sparked a significant culture change. By encouraging input from all team members and breaking down traditional hierarchies, Pronovost created an atmosphere where everyone felt accountable for patient safety and empowered to take action. The outcomes were truly remarkable.

At Johns Hopkins, the rate of CLABSIs in the ICU decreased to nearly zero. When the approach was implemented in over 100 intensive care units in Michigan, the impact was seen on a larger scale: Within just 18 months, the initiative prevented over 1500 infections, saved more than 1500 lives, and cut health care costs by almost $200 million [18].

However, what truly made this initiative revolutionary was not just the checklist. It was the readiness of a doctor to admit, "Maybe I don't have all the answers. Maybe I need to listen more attentively." Pronovost didn't just advocate for an intervention—he exemplified a new form of leadership grounded in modesty, collaborative decision-making, and reverence for every voice in the care team.

He reflected later: "We often assume that if something goes wrong, someone must be at fault. But what we discovered is that safety is not about striving harder. It's about establishing systems that facilitate doing the right thing."

His journey illustrates the power of integrating feedback into the very essence of care provision. When physicians embrace a culture of listening—particularly to those whose perspectives are often overlooked—transformative change becomes achievable. Dr. Pronovost didn't just lower infection rates; he reinstated dignity and trust in a broken system and proved humility is not a weakness in medicine—it's a driver of progress.

- **Practicing Gratitude and Presence**

Humility shines through in a medical provider's capacity to show gratitude and be fully present. When providers focus entirely on the patient in front of them, it conveys genuine care and respect. In the hectic health care landscape, it's easy to get sidetracked or feel rushed, but a humble provider makes it a priority to connect with patients on a personal level. Practicing gratitude means recognizing the hard work of everyone, from nursing staff to administrative teams, and expressing appreciation for their contributions. This combination of gratitude and presence enhances the medical provider-patient relationship and fosters a more positive work atmosphere for everyone.

In the mid-twentieth century, few illnesses instilled more fear than poliomyelitis. Polio was not only deadly but cruel—paralyzing children, forcing them into iron lungs and leaving families devastated. At the height of the epidemic in the early 1950s, over 50,000 cases were reported each year in the United States alone. Public panic was palpable. Parks emptied, pools were drained, and a generation of parents lived in daily terror that their child could be next.

During a time of great worry, Dr. Jonas Salk stood out not as a flashy hero but as a quiet, thoughtful doctor and scientist who valued humility, presence, and gratitude just as much as his groundbreaking research. His motivation was not fame or fortune but a genuine desire to alleviate suffering. He believed hope is found in dreams, imagination, and the bravery to turn dreams into reality. Dr. Salk's laboratory at the University of Pittsburgh was at the forefront of a monumental public health initiative, but he never saw it as solely his achievement. He constantly stressed the collaborative effort behind the discoveries, expressing gratitude to the researchers, technicians, volunteers, and the families involved in what became the largest medical field trial in history.

Salk was known not only for his scientific expertise but also for his exceptional ability to connect with people. He showed deep empathy toward parents, children, and health care workers affected by polio, visiting wards, listening to patients, and acknowledging the efforts of nurses and staff. Even after the successful vaccine trial, he focused on the millions of children who would benefit rather than personal glory. He walked alone for hours, reflecting on the families, patients, and everyone involved in the breakthrough.

A significant moment defined his legacy, not in science but in his character. When questioned about patenting the vaccine, which could have brought him immense wealth, Salk humbly replied, "There is no patent. Could you patent the sun?" This response was not a show; it was the sincere reply of a man who viewed the vaccine as more than a commodity but a generous offering to humanity. He considered the vaccine a collaborative effort, achieved through shared sacrifices and collective determination. By choosing not to patent it, he expressed profound gratitude and a desire to give back to the world that had entrusted him with the crucial duty of healing.

Dr. Jonas Salk's life shows us that humility in medicine is more about presence than modesty. It's about being fully engaged with those we serve, recognizing those who support us, and showing gratitude every step of the way. Deep and sincere gratitude can be a form of leadership, and being present is a powerful way to heal, especially in uncertain times [17, 19].

In 2017, Dr. David Shulkin, a former US Secretary of Veterans Affairs and a respected physician, showcased the incredible impact of gratitude and presence in health care. He worked diligently to enhance their health care experiences throughout his career dedicated to serving veterans. What truly distinguished him was his heartfelt connection with patients and his sincere appreciation for the health care team surrounding him.

While he was Secretary of Veterans Affairs, Dr. Shulkin regularly visited hospitals and medical centers, making a point to be present and acknowledge not just the veterans but also the doctors, nurses, and administrative staff who tirelessly cared for them. During a visit to the VA Medical Center in Washington, DC, he took a moment from his busy schedule to walk through the hospital wards and interact with veterans in their rooms. His purpose was not merely to reassure them about the health care system but to genuinely listen to their stories, inquire about their needs, and express gratitude for their service and patience within the system.

In one particularly moving encounter, Dr. Shulkin sat down with a veteran undergoing treatment for several months. After hearing about the veteran's experience, Dr. Shulkin acknowledged the challenges the veteran had faced and expressed gratitude for their strength and perseverance. He then thanked the medical team for caring for the patient. He emphasized that their hard work and dedication made a tangible difference in the lives of the veterans they served. This act of gratitude was not a casual remark—it was an intentional acknowledgment of their contributions, reinforcing the value of every team member.

Dr. Shulkin's approach to practicing gratitude and being fully present with his patients and staff created an atmosphere of respect and trust. He understood the importance of showing appreciation for those who worked on the front lines of care and ensured they felt seen and valued. His presence was not only therapeutic for the patients but also for the health care staff, who often felt overworked and underappreciated in a system that struggled to meet the needs of all veterans.

Dr. Shulkin's efforts highlight how important it is for health care providers to practice gratitude and be present with their patients and teams. This approach fosters a positive environment where people feel heard, respected, and motivated to give their best. His legacy as a leader in veteran care is marked by his ability to connect with people on a human level, showing that the smallest gestures of gratitude can have a profound impact on both the patient and the health care system [21].

In medicine, humility is not merely a soft skill but a fundamental competency. The stories and practices shared here show humility is not about diminishing oneself but uplifting others: listening attentively, involving others in decisions, admitting mistakes, welcoming feedback, and showing sincere appreciation. A humble health care provider understands healing is a collaborative process that thrives on trust, teamwork, and being present. Whether it's Dr. Verghese's attentive listening, Dr. Gawande's dedication to collaboration, Dr. Goldman's openness about imperfections, Dr. Hanna-Attisha's courage in seeking community input, Dr. Pronovost's openness to frontline perspectives, or the gracious demeanor of Drs Salk and Shulkin—these examples highlight a profound truth: humility enhances care. It encourages patients to be active partners, teams to work cohesively, and systems to operate more safely. In the fast-paced world of health care, humility is not a luxury but a potent, enduring force that connects us through our shared humanity.

## Conclusion

In conclusion, humility is an essential trait in health care that directly contributes to better patient care and stronger professional relationships. It involves recognizing one's limitations, embracing learning opportunities, and prioritizing patient well-being over personal ego. Humility fosters trust, collaboration, and open communication among health care providers and patients. It also encourages the acknowledgment of mistakes, the acceptance of feedback, and the practice of gratitude. Ultimately, humility enhances the quality of care and supports a more effective, compassionate health care environment.

**Take-Home Points**

- Humility in health care improves patient care by fostering trust and collaboration.
- Acknowledging one's limitations allows for continuous learning and growth.
- Prioritizing patient needs over ego strengthens the doctor-patient relationship.
- Admitting mistakes and seeking feedback leads to better outcomes and personal growth.
- Practicing gratitude enhances the health care environment and team dynamics.

## References


1. Apgar V. A proposal for a new method of evaluation of the newborn infant. Curr Res Anesth Analg. 1953;32(4):260–7. https://www.ncbi.nlm.nih.gov/pubmed/13083014
2. Awdish R. In shock: my journey from death to recovery and the redemptive power of hope. New York: St. Martin's Press; 2017a.
3. Awdish RL. A view from the edge – creating a culture of caring. N Engl J Med. 2017b;376(1):7–9. https://doi.org/10.1056/NEJMp1614078.
4. Best M, Neuhauser D. Ignaz Semmelweis and the birth of infection control. Qual Saf Health Care. 2004;13(3):233–4. https://doi.org/10.1136/qhc.13.3.233.
5. Bishop PJ. Evolution of the stethoscope. J R Soc Med. 1980;73(6):448–56. https://doi.org/10.1177/014107688007300611.
6. Choudry M, Stead TS, Mangal RK, Ganti L. The history and evolution of the stethoscope. Cureus. 2022;14(8):e28171. https://doi.org/10.7759/cureus.28171.
7. Codell Carter K, Carter BR. Childbed fever: a scientific biography of Ignaz Semmelweis. Revised ed. London: Routledge; 2005.
8. David L, Dumitrascu DL. The bicentennial of the stethoscope: a reappraisal. Clujul Med. 2017;90(3):361–3. https://doi.org/10.15386/cjmed-821
9. Ditum S. A second medical opinion is a right, not a privilege. Sunday Times. 2024. https://www.thetimes.com/comment/columnists/article/second-medical-opinion-martha-rule-privilege-nd8zpxtr5?utm_source=chatgpt.com&region=global
10. Elashmawy A, Haq A, Federico A, Chokr M, Bazzi AJ. Scoring for life: the legacy of Virginia Apgar in neonatal medicine. Cureus. 2024;16(9):e69281. https://doi.org/10.7759/cureus.69281.
11. Gallagher TH, Garbutt JM, Waterman AD, Flum DR, Larson EB, Waterman BM, Dunagan WC, Fraser VJ, Levinson W. Choosing your words carefully: how physicians would disclose harmful medical errors to patients. Arch Intern Med. 2006;166(15):1585–93. https://doi.org/10.1001/archinte.166.15.1585.
12. Gawande A. The checklist manifesto: how to get things right. New York: Metropolitan Books; 2009.
13. Goldman B. Doctors make mistakes. Can we talk about that? Ted; 2010. https://www.youtube.com/watch?v=iUbfRzxNy20.
14. Goldman B. The night shift. New York: HarperCollins Publishers; 2011.
15. Goldman B. The power of kindness: why empathy is essential in everyday life. Toronto: HarperCollins Publishers; 2018.
16. Hanna-Attisha M. What the eyes don't see: a story of crisis, resistance, and hope in an American City. New York: One World; 2018.
17. Oshinsky DM. Polio: an American story. Oxford: Oxford University Press; 2005.

18. Pronovost P, Needham D, Berenholtz S, Sinopoli D, Chu H, Cosgrove S, Sexton B, Hyzy R, Welsh R, Roth G, Bander J, Kepros J, Goeschel C. An intervention to decrease catheter-related bloodstream infections in the ICU. N Engl J Med. 2006;355(26):2725–32. https://doi.org/10.1056/NEJMoa061115.
19. Salik J. Man unfolding. New York: Harper & Row; 1972.
20. Sheffield T. Man needed double leg and arm amputations after routine kidney stone surgery: 'he was so independent'. People. 2025. https://people.com/man-needed-double-leg-and-arm-amputations-after-routine-kidney-stone-surgery-8788497?utm_source=chatgpt.com
21. Shulkin D. It shouldn't be this hard to serve your country: our broken government and the plight of veterans. New York: PublicAffairs; 2019.
22. Verghese A. Cutting for stone. New York: Vintage; 2009.
23. Wu AW. Medical error: the second victim. The doctor who makes the mistake needs help too. BMJ. 2000;320(7237):726–7. https://doi.org/10.1136/bmj.320.7237.726.

# 3 Mindfulness

Dr. Emily Carter was at her desk, reviewing patient charts as noon approached. The hospital was alive with its usual hustle and bustle—phones ringing, nurses hurrying through the corridors, and the faint sound of a code blue alert in another area. She was a bit behind schedule, and the need to catch up felt heavy on her shoulders.

Her next patient, Mrs. Evelyn Grant, a 68-year-old woman recently diagnosed with metastatic lung cancer, was patiently waiting in Exam Room 3. Dr. Carter quickly reviewed the notes: "Patient seeking options for palliative care versus aggressive treatment. Reports increased shortness of breath and fatigue." She took a deep breath, knowing she had another tough conversation ahead on this already challenging day.

As Dr. Carter stepped into the room, she spotted Mrs. Grant seated in a chair, her hands firmly holding the edges of her floral skirt. Despite the weariness in her eyes, there was a glimmer of hope as she searched for something unspoken. Emily began sharing the clinical details: the latest laboratory results, imaging findings, and possible treatment options. She explained the prognosis clearly, her voice steady yet somewhat distant, as her thoughts drifted to the growing list of tasks ahead of her.

"Dr Carter," Mrs. Grant gently interrupted, her voice trembling, "Do you think there's still time for me to see my granddaughter graduate?"

The question lingered in the air. For a brief moment, Emily hesitated. She realized she had been so focused on presenting the facts and checking off boxes that she hadn't acknowledged the woman before her—the grandmother, the fighter, the person holding onto the hope of experiencing one more family milestone.

Taking a deep breath, Dr. Carter settled in, making eye contact with Mrs. Grant. She allowed a moment of silence to envelop them before gently asking, "Can you tell me about your granddaughter?" A warm smile spread across Mrs. Grant's face as she shared stories about her 17-year-old, who was getting ready for high school graduation. Tears filled her eyes as she expressed her dreams and worries.

In that moment, Dr. Carter sensed a change. The rush of the day faded away, replaced by a deep connection. She realized she wasn't just addressing a medical


F. Aziz, *The Healing Art of Connecting with Patients*,
https://doi.org/10.1007/978-3-032-03624-7_3

issue but buying a person. They spent the next 20 min discussing treatment options and how to cherish the time Mrs. Grant had ahead.

When the conversation ended, Mrs. Grant shared her appreciation, her voice calm and determined. "Thank you for listening," she said. "I feel like I'm more than just another name on a list." As Dr. Carter stepped out of the room, she understood that being genuinely present—both physically and emotionally—had changed the experience. It wasn't solely about the medicine; it was about the human connection that accompanied it. That day, Emily promised to engage in each patient interaction with mindfulness, acknowledging that the gift of presence could be as impactful as any treatment she recommended.

In today's fast-paced and demanding health care environment, being fully engaged during patient interactions can seem more like a luxury than a must-have. However, mindfulness—the art of being aware and present in the moment—can genuinely change how we provide patient care. It connects the technical skills of health care with the essential human touch that is fundamental to medicine.

But sometimes, the call to be fully present arises not in the quiet of a clinic room, but in moments of chaos—when presence becomes an act of courage.

On April 15, 2013, thousands gathered in Boston to celebrate Patriots' Day and cheer on runners at the Boston Marathon. The atmosphere was joyful—families lined the streets, children held handmade signs, and volunteers handed out water as runners neared the finish line. Among the participants was Dr. Natalie Stavas, a pediatrician at Boston Children's Hospital, running the marathon for the first time to raise money for child advocacy programs.

But at 2:49 PM, everything took a turn. Two homemade bombs went off near the finish line, tragically claiming three lives and injuring over 260 others. Shrapnel scattered through the air, smoke filled the street, and screams filled the atmosphere as panic spread and chaos ensued. Most people instinctively fled the scene.

Dr. Stavas took a different approach. Still wearing her running shoes and bib number, she dashed toward the smoke. Without any protective gear or awareness, she crossed police barriers and hurried into the chaos. The first person she saw was a man with a severely injured leg. Without hesitation, she kneeled, removed her belt, and fashioned a makeshift tourniquet to help stem the blood flow. She stayed by his side, looking into his eyes and speaking soothingly as she applied pressure. "I'm a doctor," she reassured him. "I'm here with you. We're going to get through this together."

Dr. Stavas moved from one person to another, collaborating with first responders to stabilize injuries, ensure airways were clear, and provide comfort amidst the chaos. What kept her steady in such a terrifying situation? In later interviews, she shared it boiled down to one key aspect: presence. "I concentrated on the next breath," she mentioned. "I kept reminding myself to stay in the moment, not to get lost in the noise or fear. Just be here. Right now."

Later on, she would think back on how her medical training equipped her for crises, but it was her practice of mindful presence—being aware, calm, and connected—that enabled her to respond effectively and compassionately amid chaos.

"You can't control what's happening around you," she shared. "But you can control how you respond to it. That's where the real power lies."

Dr. Stavas was honored as the 2013 Bostonian of the Year by *The Boston Globe* for her bravery. Her actions became a symbol not only of courage but also of clarity under pressure—showing mindfulness in medicine goes beyond self-care; it's about being fully present when people need support the most [3].

This chapter will explore mindfulness in clinical practice and its significant effects on patients and health care providers. We will examine scientific research, practical strategies, and real-life stories to see how mindfulness can improve communication, build trust, and enhance decision-making.

## Defining Mindfulness in Medical Practice

Mindfulness in medical practice is all about intentionally fostering full awareness, presence, and focus during interactions with patients and while making clinical decisions. It encourages health care providers to fully engage with their patients, their surroundings, and themselves, all while being present in the moment without judgment.

At its essence, mindfulness is about purposeful attention. For health care providers, this means genuinely listening to what a patient says, picking up on subtle nonverbal signals, and responding thoughtfully instead of impulsively. It goes beyond just the patient interaction, involving a conscious awareness of one's emotions, biases, and thought processes that can affect the quality of care.

Mindfulness in medicine is both a mental discipline and a practice. It takes deliberate effort to navigate the distractions of modern health care—like time constraints, electronic health records, and multitasking—and to prioritize being present. This commitment enhances care quality by nurturing empathy, improving communication, and supporting better clinical decisions.

Dr. Ron Epstein, a prominent advocate for mindfulness in medicine, describes it as "attentiveness to the ordinary and extraordinary moments of patient care." This level of attentiveness benefits patients and helps medical providers manage stress, alleviate burnout, and find fulfillment in their work. By embracing mindfulness, medical practice becomes a harmonious blend of scientific precision and compassionate connection [8].

## Dr. William Osler and the Practice of "Aequanimitas"

In the late nineteenth and early twentieth centuries, Dr. William Osler became a prominent figure in medicine. Often called the "Father of Modern Medicine," Osler transformed medical education by focusing on bedside teaching, patient-centered care, and the blend of science with the art of healing. Beyond his clinical skills, Osler was a thoughtful philosopher of medicine who highlighted the significance of mindfulness—referring to it as "equanimity" and "calm presence"—in managing the complexities of patient care.

One of his most famous speeches, *Aequanimitas*, given to graduating medical students in 1889, beautifully sums up his philosophy. Google search reveals that the term "aequanimitas," derived from Latin, refers to equanimity, which is the ability to remain calm and balanced even in stressful situations. For Osler, this quality was crucial for dealing with the emotional hurdles of medical practice and delivering compassionate and effective care. His insights are a timeless reminder of how mindfulness—being fully present and calm—can enhance the medical provider-patient relationship.

Osler's approach to medicine was all about being fully present. Renowned for his calm demeanor, he often sat quietly by a patient's bedside, paying close attention to every detail and listening intentionally. His soothing presence created an environment where patients felt valued and understood, allowing for the discovery of subtle clinical insights.

Dr. William Osler once demonstrated his clinical expertise and compassion by successfully diagnosing a challenging case of endocarditis. His thorough examination and careful observation identified subtle signs that others had missed, ultimately making a rare diagnosis. Osler's dedication to patient care extended beyond diagnosis, as he supported the patients and their families throughout the complex process. This case showcased Osler's diagnostic abilities and emphasized the importance of empathy and human connection in medicine.

Osler often reflected on experiences like this, stressing that being fully present—rather than rushing to conclusions or getting sidetracked by outside pressures—was essential for practicing good medicine. This mindful approach to care became a defining characteristic of his practice and teachings.

One of Osler's central ideas was the importance of "living in the present moment." He recognized that physicians often wrestled with past mistakes or future uncertainties, which could cloud their judgment and erode their capacity to care effectively. Focusing on the here and now, Osler believed physicians could provide better care and find greater fulfillment in their work.

Osler modeled this philosophy throughout his career. Despite his many accomplishments and accolades, he remained profoundly humble and attuned to the humanity of his patients. His ability to connect with people, not just treat diseases, set him apart as a clinician and teacher [2, 5, 15].

## Dr. Helen Taussig and the Blueprint for Modern Pediatric Cardiology

In the mid-twentieth century, Dr. Helen Taussig, fondly known as the "Mother of Pediatric Cardiology," made remarkable strides in tackling congenital heart defects through careful observation and innovative ideas. Her pioneering development of the first effective surgical treatment of "blue baby syndrome" saved countless lives and transformed the field of pediatric medicine.

Before the 1940s, children born with cyanotic heart defects—marked by oxygen-poor blood that gives the skin a bluish hue—faced a grim fate. While doctors could identify the condition, they had no treatments available. These defects often stemmed from structural issues in the heart, like the tetralogy of Fallot, which hindered proper blood oxygenation.

Dr. Helen Taussig, a physician at Johns Hopkins, was passionate about finding a solution. Despite her partial deafness, she was celebrated for her remarkable attentiveness and diagnostic abilities. She had a unique way of "listening" to a patient's heart through her fingers, picking up on details that others might miss. Her keen focus on her patients led her to theorize that altering blood flow could enhance oxygenation in infants with cyanosis. She proposed a groundbreaking idea of creating a bypass to allow more oxygen-rich blood to reach the body. This was a bold concept when cardiac surgery was just developing.

Teaming up with Dr. Alfred Blalock, a surgeon, and Vivien Thomas, an innovative surgical technician at Johns Hopkins Hospital, they crafted the first procedure to treat cyanotic heart disease: the Blalock-Taussig shunt. This surgery established an artificial link between a major artery and the pulmonary artery, boosting blood flow to the lungs and improving oxygen levels. In 1944, they successfully performed the first surgery on a child with blue baby syndrome. The results were remarkable, significantly reducing the child's cyanosis. This success heralded the dawn of modern pediatric cardiac surgery.

Dr. Taussig's thoughtful approach was key to her achievements. Her ability to connect patient symptoms with anatomical insights and creative solutions transformed pediatric cardiology. Her commitment to fully engaging with her patients—listening to their stories and understanding their physiology—showcases the power of mindfulness in health care.

Beyond her surgical contributions, Taussig also championed children's health on a larger scale, notably raising awareness about the risks of thalidomide, a drug associated with birth defects, in the 1960s. Her legacy lives on in the many lives saved due to her groundbreaking work. Taussig's journey illustrates how mindful observation and a focus on patient needs can drive significant advancements in medical care. Her story emphasizes the value of teamwork and the bravery to innovate when faced with daunting challenges [1, 9, 19].

## Origin of Mindfulness and Its Adaptation in the Modern Era

Mindfulness is a wonderful practice and philosophy that traces back to ancient traditions, especially Buddhism. The term comes from the Pali word *Sati*, meaning "awareness" or "attentiveness." In Buddhist teachings, mindfulness is a key part of the Eightfold Path, which guides ethical living and mental practices aimed at achieving enlightenment. It encourages us to be aware of the present moment while embracing our experiences with a non-judgmental and accepting mindset.

The foundational text, *Satipaṭṭhāna Sutta*, highlights mindfulness practices that concentrate on four key areas: the body, feelings, the mind, and mental objects.

These practices are designed to enhance self-awareness, emotional balance, and clarity. Throughout the centuries, mindfulness has evolved within various traditions, including Theravāda, Zen, and Tibetan Buddhism, where meditation has been essential in nurturing a calm and focused mind [18].

We can also find similar principles in other traditions, such as ancient Stoicism, which focused on emotional regulation and self-awareness, and Hindu practices like yoga and Vedanta, which employ meditative techniques to foster inner peace. Christian mysticism and Islamic Sufism also incorporate contemplative practices that resonate with mindfulness, showcasing its universal significance across different cultures and philosophies.

Mindfulness made its way into modern medicine and psychology thanks to Jon Kabat-Zinn's pioneering work in the late twentieth century. As a molecular biologist and meditator, Kabat-Zinn saw how mindfulness could help tackle today's health issues. In 1979, he established the Mindfulness-Based Stress Reduction (MBSR) program at the University of Massachusetts Medical School. This eight-week program blends mindfulness meditation, yoga, and body awareness to assist individuals in managing stress, chronic pain, and illness. By focusing on the secular and evidence-based aspects of mindfulness, Kabat-Zinn opened the door for many people to benefit from it, separating it from its spiritual roots. This transition marked the start of mindfulness being recognized as a scientifically supported therapeutic tool. Other approaches, like Mindfulness-Based Cognitive Therapy (MBCT), were introduced to build on this groundwork. Developed by Zindel Segal, Mark Williams, and John Teasdale, MBCT combines mindfulness with cognitive-behavioral techniques to help prevent depression relapse [11, 14].

Mindfulness is especially important for health care providers who face unique challenges in their roles. The high levels of stress, emotional fatigue, and burnout that come from long hours, complex decisions, and the emotional demands of caring for patients can be overwhelming. Mindfulness offers a valuable way to cope with these pressures while improving clinical performance and personal well-being. Being fully present during patient interactions allows medical providers to listen actively, pick up on nonverbal signals, and respond with empathy.

## Practical Techniques for Integrating Mindfulness in Medicine

Incorporating mindfulness doesn't mean medical providers have to meditate for long hours. Taking small, practical steps can make a big difference in clinical practice. Some of these mindful techniques are summarized in Table 3.1.

### The Stop Technique

The STOP technique is a simple mindfulness exercise that helps health care professionals refresh their mental state under challenging situations. Derived from MBSR

**Table 3.1** Mindfulness practices in clinical settings

| Technique | Description | When to use | Benefits |
|---|---|---|---|
| STOP technique | Pause<br>Take a breath<br>Observe<br>Proceed with intention | Before difficult conversations<br>During emotional or high-stress moments | Reduces reactivity<br>Enhances decision-making<br>Calms the nervous system |
| Mindful listening | Focused<br>Non-judgmental listening with eye contact and emotional presence | During patient interviews<br>Breaking bad news<br>Team discussions | Builds trust<br>Improves patient satisfaction<br>Enhances empathy |
| Box breathing | Inhale<br>Hold<br>Exhale<br>Pause<br>(each for 4 s) in a rhythmic pattern | Before high-pressure procedures<br>During emotional fatigue or overwhelm | Reduces anxiety<br>Regulates heart rate<br>Improves clarity and focus |
| Mindful touch | Intentional<br>Gentle touch with awareness of patient's comfort and boundaries | Comforting patients<br>Adjusting position or blankets<br>End-of-life care | Boosts oxytocin<br>Conveys compassion<br>Calms patients and providers |

programs created by Jon Kabat-Zinn, this method is well-known for its ease and impact in high-pressure settings [12, 14].

The acronym stands for:

- **S**—Stop what you are doing.
- **T**—Take a deep breath.
- **O**—Observe your thoughts, feelings, and surroundings without judgment.
- **P**—Proceed with focus and intention.

Research indicates that mindfulness practices, such as STOP, can activate the parasympathetic nervous system, leading to relaxation and increased clarity. This response helps reduce the "fight or flight" reaction, enabling health care providers to transition from reactive thinking to intentional responses in critical situations [6]. A study conducted at Harvard Medical School showed that mindfulness interventions notably enhanced emotional regulation, decreased impulsive decision-making, and improved performance in high-pressure environments [14].

The STOP method is advantageous in different clinical situations where emotions run high, decisions are complex, and patient interactions are crucial. By incorporating the STOP method into their routine, health care professionals can effectively handle stress, remain calm during challenging discussions, and improve their connection with patients.

### Before Difficult Conversations

A powerful way to use the STOP technique is before sharing challenging news or discussing sensitive medical information. Health care providers often encounter emotionally charged situations when delivering difficult diagnoses or exploring treatment options with patients and families. Practicing the STOP technique beforehand helps providers pause, gather their thoughts, and compose themselves before these crucial conversations.

This pause is crucial as it prevents providers from rushing through crucial details or appearing detached. By pausing, reflecting on their emotions, and regaining composure, medical providers can approach these discussions with a sense of calm and clarity, ultimately enhancing the delivery of information and building patient trust.

For instance, in a palliative care scenario, a physician paused to use the STOP technique before discussing a terminal diagnosis with a family. This brief pause allowed the doctor to calm her mind, listen attentively to the family's concerns, and transition from a clinical explanation to a compassionate dialogue. This intentional pause facilitated a more empathetic conversation, enabling the family to share their anxieties and find comfort beyond medical facts.

### During Times of Heightened Emotions

Emotions can run high in health care environments, particularly in conflict, stress, or frustration. When faced with upset patients, distressed family members, or impatient colleagues, health care providers may naturally react with frustration or defensiveness. Using the STOP technique during these times allows for a mindful pause, helping providers respond calmly instead of impulsively.

By taking a moment to acknowledge their own emotions without judgment, providers can manage their feelings and consciously opt for a more compassionate and measured reply. This mindful approach often reduces tension and enhances communication.

For instance, imagine a nurse overwhelmed during a tense interaction with a distraught family member. Applying the STOP technique, she paused to observe her frustration without judgment, regaining her composure. This brief pause enabled her to reply with empathy rather than defensiveness, resolving the conflict and steering the conversation toward mutual understanding and support.

### Between Patient Encounters

Resetting focus between patient encounters is vital for staying present and preventing emotional exhaustion. Health care providers often carry the mental and emotional burden of prior interactions into the next visit, which may hinder their ability to engage fully. By pausing mindfully, medical providers can release lingering stress from past conversations, quiet anxious thoughts, and get ready to connect meaningfully with their next patient. This practice fosters a feeling of mental "closure" after each visit, reducing the emotional strain that can lead to burnout.

The STOP technique is a valuable tool in today's busy medical world. Teaching health care professionals to pause, breathe, and observe without judgment empowers them to respond with calm focus instead of reacting impulsively. Integrating STOP into daily routines helps health care providers balance medical accuracy with compassion, enhancing their relationship with patients and protecting their mental health.

## Mindful Listening

Mindful listening is a fundamental mindfulness technique that dramatically improves communication in health care environments. By promoting focused attention and empathy, mindful listening enables health care professionals to gain a deeper insight into their patients' worries, leading to better diagnosis accuracy, building trust, and improving patient results. Engaging in mindful listening can turn ordinary discussions into valuable exchanges that support patients and provide solace in times of vulnerability.

To effectively practice mindful listening, health care providers can use the following techniques:

- **Maintain Eye Contact:** Providers show presence and attentiveness by maintaining eye contact, indicating the speaker's words are valued. In clinical settings, intentional eye contact fosters a sense of trust and safety, enabling patients to express themselves openly.
- **Minimize Internal Distractions:** Health care professionals should consciously set aside internal distractions, such as anxious thoughts or clinical concerns, to focus fully on the patient's words and nonverbal cues. This helps in understanding the emotional context behind the patient's concerns.
- **Respond with Thoughtful Pauses:** Mindful listeners use pauses to allow patients to express their thoughts fully. These pauses create room for reflection, making patients feel respected and acknowledged. It also helps providers respond more empathetically and accurately.

In health care settings, it is crucial to practice mindful listening, especially when patients are feeling vulnerable or overwhelmed. Health care professionals who listen carefully and stay engaged can build better relationships with their patients, creating a supportive environment for them to communicate essential information.

Mindful listening is a valuable and straightforward method that enhances health care communication. Through promoting presence, empathy, and curiosity, mindful listening improves patient-provider relationships, boosts diagnostic accuracy, and enhances patient outcomes. Dr. Rachel Naomi Remen aptly said, "Listening is the oldest and perhaps the most powerful healing tool. When we listen, we offer ourselves" [16].

## Box Breathing for Emotional Regulation

Box breathing, also called square breathing, is a straightforward yet effective breathing technique that helps manage emotions, lower stress levels, and enhance mental focus. It is a popular method utilized by Navy SEALs, emergency responders, and individuals in high-stress situations to stay composed and focused during times of intense pressure.

The technique consists of four simple steps, each lasting for 4 s:

- Step 1: Breathe in slowly and deeply for 4 s, filling the lungs while expanding the abdomen.
- Step 2: Hold your breath for 4 s, keeping your muscles calm and relaxed.
- Step 3: Breathe out slowly and fully for 4 s, releasing all tension as you exhale.
- Step 4: Pause for 4 s before starting the cycle again.

Box breathing is a powerful technique that can help you stay calm and in control during stressful situations. This rhythmic breathing pattern activates the parasympathetic nervous system, which counteracts the body's stress response. By practicing box breathing, medical providers can regulate their heart rate, lower cortisol levels, and enhance oxygen exchange in their bodies. Scientific studies have shown that this controlled breathing exercise stimulates the vagus nerve, improving heart rate variability and emotional regulation. Mastering box breathing can increase resilience to stress and boost cognitive performance in high-pressure scenarios [13, 17].

Box breathing can benefit health care providers in emotionally intense situations like emergency care, difficult patient conversations, or high-stakes clinical decision-making. For example, before performing an emergency procedure, a trauma surgeon found relief by using box breathing to calm her mind. This intentional breathing practice helped stabilize her heart rate, reduce anxiety, and enhance focus, enabling her to work precisely under pressure. To combat emotional fatigue during a long shift, an ICU nurse incorporated box breathing into her breaks to reset her nervous system. Five minutes of this mindful technique left her feeling more centered, calmer, and better equipped to connect empathetically with her patients.

Box breathing is a valuable mindfulness technique that can help health care providers stay calm, focused, and emotionally balanced. This method improves mental clarity and stabilizes the nervous system, enhancing clinical performance and personal well-being. In demanding health care settings, box breathing is a proven and practical way for professionals to manage stress in the moment.

## Mindful Touch in Patient Care

Mindful touch is a powerful yet often overlooked aspect of compassionate patient care. For health care providers in direct patient care roles, simple gestures—such as placing a hand on a patient's shoulder, adjusting a blanket with intention, or offering a comforting touch during moments of anxiety—can create profound connections that enhance trust and emotional well-being.

Studies show that purposeful, kind touch can trigger the production of oxytocin, known as the "bonding hormone," enhancing feelings of safety, trust, and connection. Gentle touch also engages the parasympathetic nervous system, decreasing cortisol levels and reducing heart rate, leading to a peaceful state for both the individual receiving touch and the one providing it [4, 10].

Mindful touch can enhance connection and provide comfort in patient care in various ways:

- **During Sensitive Conversations:** A gentle touch on the patient's hand or shoulder before delivering challenging news can create a calming presence, fostering trust and emotional stability.
- **In Bedside Assistance:** Adjusting a patient's blanket or pillow with awareness demonstrates compassion and attentiveness, particularly for patients who may feel isolated or fearful.
- **During Painful Situations:** Holding a patient's hand during a painful procedure or moments of anxiety can ease discomfort and provide emotional support.

For example, a hospice nurse caring for a terminally ill patient noticed the patient's discomfort despite minimal verbal communication. The nurse offered reassurance and comfort by placing a warm hand on the patient's arm while adjusting the pillow. The patient's breathing slowed, and his facial tension visibly eased—a silent yet powerful moment of connection.

## Mindful Touch and Cultural Sensitivity

It's crucial for health care providers to consider cultural, personal, and situational boundaries when using touch. Asking for permission before physical contact can help show respect and build trust, especially for patients with preferences or histories that make them uncomfortable with touch.

- **Take a Moment Before Reaching Out:** Before touching a patient, pause to ensure the gesture is caring and suitable.
- **Be Fully Engaged:** Concentrate on the patient while you touch them. This focused attention enhances the healing effect.
- **Watch for Nonverbal Signals:** Notice the patient's body language to confirm your touch is appreciated and soothing.

Mindful touch is a powerful method to convey empathy, compassion, and connection in health care. Through intentional presence and gentle touch, health care professionals can build trust, reduce anxiety, and offer emotional support to patients in difficult times. As Florence Nightingale wisely noted, "It is the unspoken things that matter most."

## Mindfulness in High-stress Situations

Health care providers frequently operate in high-pressure settings where quick decisions are essential. Practicing mindfulness equips them with important skills to remain focused and composed, enabling them to stay calm, attentive, and level-headed.

## Mindfulness During a Code Blue Situation

For example, in the chaos of a code blue, where every second counts, mindfulness enhances the ability to pause, regulate breathing, and make calculated decisions under pressure. During a particularly demanding night shift in my ICU rotation as an internal medicine resident, I was called to respond to a sudden code blue in the cardiac unit. The scene was chaotic—alarms blaring, nurses rushing to secure IV access, and other residents scrambling to interpret the telemetry data. The tension in the room was palpable, and the pressure to act quickly intensified.

As I entered the room, I felt the surge of adrenaline take hold—a familiar but unsettling sensation. My heart raced, my breathing became shallow, and my mind spun through worst-case scenarios. Amid the noise and urgency, I instinctively paused for a brief moment. I stepped back, inhaled deeply through my nose, and exhaled slowly through my mouth. That simple breath felt like hitting a mental reset button.

During that brief pause, I mentally reviewed the Advanced Cardiac Life Support (ACLS) algorithm, visualizing the crucial steps I needed to follow while also considering the hierarchy and the fact that all the nurses and residents were looking to me as a senior resident. I recalled the fundamental principle: the most important thing is to ensure high-quality chest compressions. With a clearer mind, I surveyed the situation. The patient's chest compressions were weak and irregular, so I calmly instructed a nurse to take over from the tired provider performing compressions. I kneeled beside the patient, placed my hands on their sternum, and began strong, consistent compressions. Counting silently in my mind helped me stay focused. After each compression, I reminded myself to remain in the moment and not let fear or uncertainty take over.

As the room remained tense, I maintained a calm, deliberate tone to guide the team. "Let's switch compressors every two minutes. Prepare for intubation. Can someone confirm the defibrillator pad placement?" With my mind steadier, I could prioritize clearly. When the defibrillator was ready, I instructed the team to clear the patient. "Charging… three… two… one… shock." The patient's body jolted, and the cardiac monitor briefly showed a flatline before switching to a slow rhythm. Recognizing the early signs of recovery, I instructed the team to continue compressions and administer the next round of epinephrine. The fog that had gripped the room began to clear, and gradually, the patient's pulse returned. The patient stabilized and was transferred to the cardiac ICU.

Afterward, reflecting on the experience, I realized the brief pause—a moment to breathe, reset, and ground myself—kept me calm and effective in that chaotic environment. Without it, I might have overlooked the poor-quality compressions or failed to communicate clearly with my team. That day, I learned a powerful lesson: mindful presence isn't a luxury—it's a necessity.

## Mindfulness During the Difficult Conversation

Delivering devastating news or discussing treatment limitations can be emotionally overwhelming for both the patient and the provider. Practicing mindfulness helps providers remain present, acknowledge their emotions, and respond with empathy.

During my oncology rotation as a resident, I vividly recall a young woman with metastatic cancer whose parents were struggling to grasp the gravity of her condition. Before entering the room, I stood outside the door momentarily, feeling the weight of the conversation ahead. I could sense the tension building within me—the pressure to deliver difficult news combined with my own emotions of sadness and uncertainty. Recognizing these feelings, I paused, closed my eyes, and took a slow, deliberate breath. Inhaling deeply, I told myself: Be present. Focus on what they need to hear—and how they need to feel.

When I stepped into the room, I noticed the mother gripping her daughter's hand tightly, her eyes filled with desperation. The father sat rigidly, his face pale and tense. I introduced myself, pulled up a chair, and gently said, "I know this is difficult. Can you tell me what's been most concerning to you?"

Instead of rushing to explain the diagnosis, I allowed myself to lean into their emotions, listening fully. The mother spoke first, sharing memories of her daughter's strength and their fears about the future. The father's frustration soon surfaced—he felt that previous updates had been rushed and confusing. By embracing silence and focusing on their words instead of medical facts alone, I created space for their emotions to unfold.

When I finally spoke about the prognosis, I did so calmly, pausing frequently to ensure they understood. I used explicit language, avoided medical jargon, and emphasized my commitment to supporting their daughter's comfort and dignity. By remaining mindful and present, I could navigate the conversation with compassion rather than rushing through it.

Despite the painful news, they later expressed gratitude—not just for the clarity I provided, but for the time I took to listen and connect with them as people. That experience reinforced how essential mindfulness is—not only for managing my emotions but also for creating meaningful moments of connection during some of the most complex medical conversations.

## Managing Emotional Fatigue

Long hours working during residency can be exhausting for health care workers, impacting their performance and increasing the risk of burnout. Trying mindfulness exercises such as the STOP method or box breathing between patient interactions can aid in refocusing and decreasing mental fatigue.

During my rotation in the emergency department as a first-year resident, I faced back-to-back critical cases. After a particularly difficult pediatric resuscitation, I felt emotionally depleted. My hands trembled slightly, and my mind raced with doubt—"Did I miss something? Could I have done more?"

The expressions on the child's parents' faces stayed with me—a mother quietly sobbing in the corner and a father nervously pacing. Their deep sorrow felt overwhelming, and I found it hard to move past it. As I entered the break room, I realized I needed to take a moment to regroup. My attending physician suggested I try box breathing to alleviate this emotional fatigue. I closed my eyes and began the practice: inhaling for 4 s, holding my breath for four, exhaling for four, and pausing for four. With each cycle, I visualized the tension melting away. Gradually, the heaviness in my chest eased, and my thoughts calmed. I reminded myself I had done everything possible to support that child.

After 2 min, my heart rate slowed, and my mind steadied. The knot in my chest loosened, and I felt grounded again. That brief reset allowed me to re-enter the busy floor with renewed composure and focus. Later that night, I realized the importance of those mindful pauses—not only for my well-being but for my patients, who needed me to be fully present in their care.

## Navigating Conflict with Colleagues

Residency can sometimes lead to intense interactions with colleagues when under stress. Feeling tired, under pressure, and making urgent clinical decisions can increase tensions. Mindfulness practice helps handle frustration, encourages positive conversations, and prevents conflicts from worsening.

During my residency on a particularly exhausting night shift, I was handling multiple admissions when a patient's condition deteriorated rapidly. I initiated aggressive fluid resuscitation and ordered urgent labs. The following day, during handoff, a senior colleague challenged my decision-making in front of the entire team.

His tone was sharp, and his frustration was evident. "Why didn't you escalate care earlier? The patient could've been transferred sooner!" His words stung, and I felt the immediate instinct to defend myself. My heart pounded, and I felt a flush of frustration rising.

At that moment, I caught myself. I paused, took a slow breath, and consciously softened my posture. Instead of reacting defensively, I said, "Can you walk me through your concerns? I want to make sure I understand."

That brief pause shifted the energy in the room. His voice steadied as he explained his perspective—that earlier consultation with the ICU might have improved outcomes. As I listened, I realized we shared the same goal: ensuring the best possible care for our patients. I helped redirect the conversation toward learning rather than blame by staying calm and inviting dialogue.

Afterward, my colleague approached me privately. "I'm sorry for how I came across earlier," he admitted. "I know you were under a lot of pressure last night." That conversation reinforced that mindfulness isn't just about staying calm for myself—it's also a powerful way to create space for understanding and collaboration in emotionally charged situations.

## Dr. Lorna Breen: The Cost of Carrying the Weight Alone

In the early days of the COVID-19 pandemic, New York City was at the heart of a global crisis. Hospitals were overwhelmed, supplies were scarce, and staff faced exhaustion, fear, and profound loss. During this turbulent time, Dr. Lorna M. Breen, the 49-year-old Medical Director of the Emergency Department at New York-Presbyterian Allen Hospital in Manhattan, stood out.

Dr. Breen embodied the qualities any hospital would admire in a leader—she was intelligent, tireless, and incredibly compassionate. With a lifelong dedication to emergency medicine, she approached patient care with a calm and focused demeanor. Even as her hospital struggled to manage an influx of critically ill COVID-19 patients, she remained steadfast on the front lines. Like many of her health care colleagues, she faced unimaginable suffering—patients passing away alone, families unable to say their goodbyes, and her teammates overwhelmed by relentless grief.

Eventually, Dr. Breen contracted COVID-19. After quarantining and recovering physically, she returned to work but still felt emotionally strained. Her colleagues noticed a difference; the woman who once mentored residents, welcomed patients warmly, and exuded quiet confidence now appeared anxious, unsettled, and withdrawn. She shared with loved ones her feelings of inadequacy, overwhelmed by the loss of life around her and believing she wasn't doing enough.

Despite this, she continued to work until she could no longer do so. Tragically, on April 26, 2020, Dr. Lorna Breen died by suicide while visiting family in Virginia, leaving the medical community in shock. She had no previous mental health issues, and her family later revealed Lorna was afraid of the professional consequences of seeking help. "She worried people would think she couldn't handle the pressure," her father, Dr. Philip Breen, noted. "But the truth is, she was the kind of doctor everyone should want—caring, capable, and dedicated."

Her tragic death illuminated an invisible epidemic within the pandemic: the mental health crisis among health care providers. It exposed how silence, stigma, and the relentless culture of self-sacrifice can strip even the most resilient physicians of their sense of worth.

In response, her family founded the Dr. Lorna Breen Heroes' Foundation, which advocates for the mental health of health care workers. Their efforts led to bipartisan legislation—the Dr. Lorna Breen Health Care Provider Protection Act, signed into law in 2022 by President Joe Biden. This federal law funds mental health resources for medical professionals, supports burnout prevention programs, and seeks to remove licensing and credentialing questions that discourage clinicians from seeking help.

Lorna's story has become an essential part of the national dialogue about clinician wellness. She is more than just a doctor who died; she represents the consequences of prioritizing others' needs over our own. Her legacy highlights the critical importance of fostering mindfulness, compassion, and humanity, not just for patients but for caregivers as well [7].

## Conclusion: Mindfulness in the Practice of Medicine

Mindfulness is an invaluable tool for health care providers, offering a pathway to deeper connections with patients, improved clinical decision-making, and enhanced emotional resilience. Clinicians can create meaningful moments beyond medical interventions by consciously pausing, listening with intent, and embracing presence. Mindfulness empowers providers to manage stress, navigate difficult conversations, and foster trust in their interactions. As health care evolves, mindfulness remains a timeless practice that enhances patient care and sustains the well-being of those dedicated to healing. Embracing mindfulness is a commitment to both professional excellence and compassionate connection.

**Take-Home Points**

- Mindfulness enhances patient care by fostering presence and empathy.
- Emotional regulation techniques improve focus and reduce stress.
- Empathy and mindful listening strengthen patient relationships.
- Historical figures like Osler and Nightingale modeled mindfulness in care.
- Simple mindfulness practices can transform daily clinical interactions.

## References


1. Blalock A. Physiopathology and surgical treatment of congenital cardiovascular defects. Harvey Lect. 1945;41:90–116. https://www.ncbi.nlm.nih.gov/pubmed/20289735
2. Bliss M. William Osler: a life in medicine. Oxford: Oxford University Press; 1999.
3. Center SR. [YouTube]. Natalie Stavas – speaker on turning chaos into courage. 2015. https://www.youtube.com/watch?v=BS25gd5UAIk
4. Coan JA, Schaefer HS, Davidson RJ. Lending a hand: social regulation of the neural response to threat. Psychol Sci. 2006;17(12):1032–9. https://doi.org/10.1111/j.1467-9280.2006.01832.x.
5. Cushing H. The life of Sir William Osler: the father of modern medicine & the first residency program. Independently published; 2023.

6. Ditto B, Eclache M, Goldman N. Short-term autonomic and cardiovascular effects of mindfulness body scan meditation. Ann Behav Med. 2006;32(3):227–34. https://doi.org/10.1207/s15324796abm3203_9.
7. Dr Lorna Breen. https://drlornabreen.org/about-lorna/
8. Epstein RM. Mindful practice. JAMA. 1999;282(9):833–9. https://doi.org/10.1001/jama.282.9.833.
9. Fye WB. W. Bruce Fye, and American cardiology: a conversation with the editor about the author and his latest book. Interview by William C. Roberts. Am J Cardiol. 1996;78(3):327–33. https://doi.org/10.1016/0002-9149(96)00321-9.
10. Hertenstein MJ, Holmes R, McCullough M, Keltner D. The communication of emotion via touch. Emotion. 2009;9(4):566–73. https://doi.org/10.1037/a0016108.
11. Kabat-Zinn J. Full catastrophe living (revised edition): using the wisdom of your body and mind to face stress, pain, and illness. New York: Bantam; 2013.
12. Kabat-Zinn J. Full catastrophe living (revised edition): using the wisdom of your body and mind to face stress, pain, and illness. New York: Bantam; 2023.
13. Lehrer PM, Gevirtz R. Heart rate variability biofeedback: how and why does it work? Front Psychol. 2014;5:756. https://doi.org/10.3389/fpsyg.2014.00756.
14. Ludwig DS, Kabat-Zinn J. Mindfulness in medicine. JAMA. 2008;300(11):1350–2. https://doi.org/10.1001/jama.300.11.1350.
15. Oslar W. Aequanimitas; with other addresses to medical students, nurses and practitioners of medicine. London: HK Lewis; 1914.
16. Remen RN. Kitchen table wisdom: stories that heal. London: Riverhead Books; 2006.
17. Russo MA, Santarelli DM, O'Rourke D. The physiological effects of slow breathing in the healthy human. Breathe (Sheff). 2017;13(4):298–309. https://doi.org/10.1183/20734735.009817.
18. Thera N. The heart of Buddhist meditation: the Buddha's way of mindfulness. San Francisco: Weiser Books; 2014.
19. Thomas V. Partners of the heart: Vivien Thomas and his work with Alfred Blalock: an autobiography. Philadelphia: University of Pennsylvania Press; 1998.

# Part II

# Building Human Connections

*Healing flows through connection—when words, tone, and presence align with intention.*

**Chapter 4: Compassion**
**Chapter 5: Communication**
**Chapter 6: Shared Decision-Making**

*Shift into outward expression—how healers show up for patients and how the human connection becomes therapeutic.*

# 4 Compassion

Dr. Emily Harris, a seasoned physician, knew the palliative care unit well. However, meeting Mrs. Linda Gray, a 68-year-old woman in the last stages of cancer, brought an unexpected insight. As morning light gently filled the room, Mrs. Gray sat up in her hospital bed, looking peacefully at the horizon from the hospital window with a calm smile.

"Good morning, Mrs Gray," Dr. Harris greeted gently as she walked in with her clipboard, ready for the usual medical conversation. Yet, the peaceful atmosphere in the room made her stop, and her typical questions slipped from her mind momentarily.

Mrs. Gray shared, "I'm simply enjoying the sunrise. It brings back memories of my garden, mornings filled with flowers and birds, surrounded by nature's beauty."

Inspired by her patient's kind demeanor, Dr. Harris chose to have a deeper conversation. She set aside her professional goals and sat beside the bed, eager to hear about Mrs. Gray's garden. "I'd be delighted to learn more," she said warmly, encouraging Mrs. Gray to share.

Mrs. Gray's eyes sparkled as she talked about her garden filled with blooming lilacs and colorful tulips. For her, the garden was more than just a bunch of plants; it was a peaceful place that made her happy and calm and an important part of life.

This sincere conversation flowed naturally, filled with genuine interest, and went beyond the usual talks between a patient and a doctor. Dr. Harris listened carefully, not just as a doctor but as a caring person. She understood this moment of connection was as healing as anything she could prescribe. Mrs. Gray's stories showed her spirit and strength, bringing comfort and a moving reminder of the deep joy in simple things.

As the conversation unfolded, Dr. Harris understood the dual nature of compassionate care. Not only did it benefit Mrs. Gray by providing her with a sense of normalcy and joy as she reminisced about cherished memories, but it also profoundly impacted Dr. Harris. This experience reignited her love for medicine and reminded her of the reasons she chose this path. She now realized more than ever that compassionate care went beyond medical treatments; it involved forming


F. Aziz, *The Healing Art of Connecting with Patients*,
https://doi.org/10.1007/978-3-032-03624-7_4

connections with patients and acknowledging their unique journeys with empathy and a genuine desire to help them. When Dr. Harris eventually rose to depart, she felt a profound satisfaction that she had rarely experienced in her usual clinical encounters. This exchange underscored the transformative influence of compassion in medicine, revealing that such moments could bridge the divide between clinical efficacy and the human aspect of illness.

In the calm setting of the hospital room, a key insight emerged: Showing kindness does more than just help with physical pain; it also lifts the spirit, improves well-being, and strengthens relationships. These moments are important for the patient and the medical providers because they bring healing, comfort, and growth. This highlights how powerful our presence can be in someone else's life.

Exploring the impact of compassionate care in history, we go back to 1807. The battlegrounds of Eylau were soaked in blood, the sounds of cannon fire echoing in the ears of soldiers and medics. During Napoleon's tumultuous campaigns, one individual stood out—not with a weapon, but by providing compassionate care and hope. Dr. Jean Dominique Larrey, Napoleon's head surgeon, swiftly navigated the battlefield. His uniform, stained with mud and blood, carried the weight of many lives. His keen eyes were fueled by a profound belief that the injured should receive prompt care, regardless of status or affiliation. Larrey transformed how wounded soldiers were treated, introducing the innovative concept of the "flying ambulance."

In times of peril, these nimble horse-drawn carriages bravely ventured into danger zones to save soldiers amidst the chaos of flying musket balls. Larrey prioritized caring for the injured based on the gravity of their wounds, regardless of their military affiliation. Whether French, Prussian, or Austrian, every life held equal value.

On a cold morning, Larrey found a young Prussian soldier with a broken leg, tears freezing on his face. Despite being an enemy, Larrey comforted him and stayed by his side during the amputation. The soldier believed Larrey's kindness and compassion saved him, not just his surgical expertise. Larrey's presence and support helped the soldier endure the pain. Larrey's compassion rippled through the ranks. Napoleon admired him deeply, calling him "the most virtuous man I have ever known." Even enemy generals respected him. After the Battle of Waterloo in 1815, when Larrey was captured by Prussian forces and faced execution, it was the same enemy soldiers—those who had heard of his mercy—who pleaded for his life to be spared.

His compassion transformed battlefield medicine and paved the way for present-day emergency response systems. Larrey also emphasized the importance of compassion in war, highlighting its strength in connecting us through our shared humanity, especially in challenging times. Larrey once wrote: "To a soldier, the loss of a limb is nothing compared to the loss of hope. A surgeon must be a technician and a source of courage." Compassionate care remains essential across time, serving as a vital link between survival and dignity, whether in a contemporary hospital setting or on a nineteenth-century battlefield [26].

Compassionate care is truly the heart and soul of effective medical practice. It's not just something we wish for; it's a crucial element that dramatically affects clinical outcomes and supports the well-being of health care providers. In the busy and sometimes overwhelming world of medicine, it's easy for compassion to be overshadowed by a focus on efficiency and technology. However, let's keep in mind the wise words of American author John Naisbitt: "The most exciting breakthroughs of the twenty-first century will not occur because of technology but because of an expanding concept of what it means to be human" [23]. This growing understanding highlights that compassion is just as vital to healing as any medical treatment, reminding us that the essence of health care is the human connection.

## A Tragic Reminder of Compassion's Importance

On February 27, 2007, a tragic accident unfolded on a treacherously snowy road in central Sweden when two buses collided shortly before 9 AM. The collision was catastrophic, claiming the lives of 6 people, seriously injuring 9, and leaving 42 others with minor injuries. The morning, which began like any other, quickly became a nightmare for those involved. The accident site was a scene of chaos, with twisted metal, shattered glass, and the anguished cries of the injured filling the cold morning air. Emergency responders rushed to the scene, battling the situation's elements and urgency. Most of the wounded were quickly transported to the University Hospital in Uppsala, a facility known for handling trauma cases. Two of the most critically injured individuals were airlifted to a Stockholm hospital in a desperate bid to save their lives. The response was swift, and from a logistical standpoint, it was considered a success given the circumstances [2].

In 2014, Doohan and colleagues contacted survivors through telephone interviews, gathering insights from 54 out of 56 individuals, including 21 women and 33 men. They explored topics such as discomfort before reaching the hospital, the absence of compassionate care, and dissatisfaction with crisis support. Even after several years, survivors vividly recalled the physical pain they experienced and the lack of compassion from emergency department nurses and health care providers. The authors highlighted how a shortage of compassion among health care professionals can significantly impact a patient's well-being, leaving lasting memories long after the traumatic event. In other words, the absence of compassion can hurt just as deeply as physical pain [7].

This study revealed a sobering truth: physical trauma is merely the tip of the iceberg. In the fast-paced realm of emergency care, where time is of the essence, one essential ingredient was noticeably missing—compassion. Survivors, already facing the chaos of pain and uncertainty, found themselves in a cold, clinical setting devoid of the human connection they desperately needed. Even with the heroic life-saving actions around them, the absence of compassion created a more profound hurt than any physical injury could inflict.

This tragic event is a stark reminder that compassion—or the lack thereof—can profoundly influence a patient's experience and recovery. In health care, this feeling often determines the patient's perception of their care and overall recovery process. Compassionate care is not merely an add-on; it is a fundamental aspect of healing that must be integrated into every interaction between health care providers and patients.

As health care systems evolve, compassion must remain central to patient care. The lessons learned from this tragedy in Sweden should remind all health care providers that their influence goes far beyond the hospital walls. It resonates in the memories of those they care for, shaping how they view health care and affecting their recovery journey. Patients and families might not recall the name or face of the doctor or nurse who assisted them during one of their most challenging moments. Still, they will never forget the comfort that health care professionals provide.

## Defining Compassion: Beyond Pity, Sympathy, and Empathy

Compassion is truly one of the most impactful forces in how we connect. It goes beyond just feeling pity or sympathy; it is about actively engaging with the struggles of others. A quick Google search reveals that the word "compassion" has its roots in the Latin term *compati*, which translates to "to suffer with."

This origin highlights the true nature of compassion: a deep, empathetic awareness of someone else's pain, paired with a heartfelt wish to help ease that suffering. Compassion encourages us to recognize suffering—whether through pity or empathy—and to take meaningful action. It transforms our understanding of someone else's challenges into a genuine commitment to make a positive change.

Unlike pity, which can be seen as a distant, almost condescending recognition of someone else's misfortune, compassion is intimate and inclusive. Pity often involves feeling sorry for someone from a position of superiority, but it lacks the drive to change the situation. It can create a barrier between the person feeling pity and suffering, reinforcing a sense of separation rather than connection.

Sympathy, while a step closer to compassion, still falls short. Sympathy allows us to feel concern for someone and perhaps share in their sorrow, but it does not necessarily require us to act. It is an emotional response acknowledging another's hardship, but it may keep us at arm's length.

Empathy brings us even closer to compassion. It enables us to feel what another person feels when walking in their shoes. Empathy creates a deep emotional resonance between individuals, fostering understanding and connection. However, even empathy, powerful as it is, can remain passive. It allows us to experience another's pain, but it does not always move us to alleviate that pain.

Compassion, on the other hand, is inherently active. It is empathy in motion. As the Dalai Lama, a famous spiritual leader, once said, "Compassion is the wish to see others free from suffering" [16]. This wish, combined with the will to act, differentiates compassion from its emotional counterparts (Fig. 4.1).

Stephen Trzeciak and Anthony Mazzarelli, in their groundbreaking book *Compassionomics*, provide a clear distinction between empathy and compassion: "Empathy is like a one-way street running toward the health care provider: detecting, processing, understanding, and even feeling the incoming emotional cues from the patient. Conversely, compassion is a street that runs in the other direction—a

**Compassion = Feeling of other's suffering + taking action to relieve that suffering**

**Fig. 4.1** Definition of compassion

responsive action toward the one who is suffering" [28]. This distinction is crucial in understanding why compassion is vital in health care settings. Empathy allows health care providers to understand and connect with their patients' emotions, and compassion compels them to take steps to ease the suffering of those under their care.

This statement highlights compassion's central role in personal fulfillment and professional excellence. In health care, the guiding principle ensures patients are treated as whole human beings, not just as cases or conditions.

Compassionate care involves recognizing the full spectrum of a patient's experience—physical, emotional, and spiritual. It means understanding that every patient is more than just a diagnosis; they are individuals with fears, hopes, and lives that extend beyond their illness. Compassion drives health care providers to look beyond the charts and symptoms, to see the person lying in the hospital bed, and to connect with them on a human level.

In practice, compassion can show up in various ways: taking a moment to explain a procedure, holding a patient's hand during tough times, offering a kind encouragement, or simply being there to listen when a patient wants to share. These seemingly small gestures can significantly enhance a patient's experience and recovery.

## Does Compassion Matter?

A key question for health care professionals often arises: *Does compassion impact patient outcomes?* The answer is a resounding *yes!* Compassion in health care is not merely a soft skill but a critical element that enhances care quality, improves patient satisfaction, and promotes well-being for patients and providers.

The release of *Compassionomics: The Revolutionary Scientific Evidence That Caring Makes a Difference* by Stephen Trzeciak and Anthony Mazzarelli has revolutionized the conversation on compassion's profound effect on clinical outcomes. Their research confirms that "caring makes a difference," showing that compassionate care can significantly improve health outcomes and reduce health care costs. Compassionate care benefits patients emotionally and leads to tangible, clinically significant results like improved treatment adherence and lower rates of hospital readmissions [28].

For example, Dr. Patch Adams, an American physician, comedian, social activist, and author, reminds us: "You treat a disease, you win, you lose. You treat a person, and I guarantee you win, no matter the outcome" [27]. This truth is echoed in a pivotal study involving diabetic patients by Hojat et al., which found that patients under the care of physicians with high empathy scores had better control of their A1c levels—56% versus 40% in patients treated by less empathetic doctors [11].

Beyond improved outcomes, compassion also mitigates the risk of malpractice claims and contributes to cost savings in health care [19]. Hippocrates once said, "Wherever the art of medicine is loved, there is also a love of humanity" [4]. When translated into compassionate care, this love can reduce expensive complications, minimize readmissions, and shorten hospital stays [20].

Dr. Francis Peabody's timeless insight encapsulates it best: "The secret of the care of the patient is in caring for the patient" [24]. Compassion fosters trust, which enhances and promotes healthier behaviors. Research consistently shows compassionate communication improves patient satisfaction, reduces pain perception, and speeds recovery [12].

## Compassion as a Defense Against Burnout

Compassionate care is beneficial for patients and a crucial defense against physician burnout, a growing concern in the medical community. Burnout among health care providers is characterized by emotional exhaustion, depersonalization, and a reduced sense of personal accomplishment. It can lead to decreased quality of care, increased medical errors, and a higher likelihood of leaving the profession. In their book *Wonder Drug: 7 Scientifically Proven Ways That Serving Others Is the Best Medicine for Yourself*, Stephen Trzeciak and Anthony Mazzarelli provide compelling evidence that compassionate care can prevent burnout and compassion fatigue among health care providers. They argue, "You don't lose anything by serving others; you only gain. Giving is a powerful therapy for the giver and give" [29].

This perspective is supported by research indicating health care providers who engage in compassionate care experience greater job satisfaction, reduced stress, and a stronger sense of purpose [5, 17, 18]. As Nelson Mandela once said, "Humility is the most important thing you should have to succeed. If you make people realize you are no threat to them, they will take no time to embrace you" [21]. This humility creates a strong foundation for a sustainable and fulfilling medical practice when combined with compassion.

Medical providers who practice compassionate care often find patient interactions more meaningful and rewarding. They develop deeper connections with their patients, enhancing the quality of care and bringing personal fulfillment. Dr. Rachel Naomi Remen observed, "The most important questions don't seem to have ready answers. But the questions themselves have a healing power when shared" [25].

I went through a challenging period in my career that opened my eyes. During my early residency years, the long hours and intense pressure wore down my initial love and dedication to medicine. I felt the signs of burnout: emotional fatigue, cynicism, and a dwindling feeling of accomplishment. Then, I had the joy of meeting a lovely elderly patient with chronic heart failure who frequently came to our clinic. Each time she visited, she brightened our day with stories about her grandchildren and her experiences as a schoolteacher, often bringing us delicious homemade treats. Her kindness and gratitude for the care she received were truly uplifting. Despite her frailty and the challenges of her illness, she always focused on what she could offer to others, radiating positivity and strength through her physical struggles.

One day, she noticed how tired I was and, taking my hand, expressed her gratitude for my commitment. She shared that our conversations and the care I offered not only helped ease her symptoms but also filled her final years with joy and comfort. Her acknowledgment of my efforts, especially when I was having difficulty seeing the worth of my work, was indeed a precious gift. It reminded me why I chose to pursue medicine—not just to treat illnesses but to make a meaningful impact on people's lives.

This experience reignited my love for medicine and imparted an important lesson about the incredible impact of compassion. It not only uplifts those on the receiving end but also rejuvenates those who give. It serves as a safeguard against the depersonalization that can come with burnout, strengthening the human connection essential in health care. Since that day, I've embraced my work with a fresh sense of purpose and dedication, realizing that every patient interaction is a chance to engage in medicine that nurtures both the patient and the caregiver.

Her impact on my life underscored the truth that compassionate care is indeed a wonder drug—not only for the patients we serve but for ourselves as health care providers, shielding us against burnout and reconnecting us with our calling.

## Steps to Cultivating Compassionate Care

Cultivating compassion in health care is a vital, ongoing process that requires intentionality, self-awareness, and a commitment to personal and professional growth. Compassion is not an innate trait one either possesses or lacks; instead, it is a skill that can be developed and refined through practice and reflection. In the demanding world of health care, where providers are often stretched thin by the pressures of time, resource limitations, and emotional challenges, fostering compassion is essential to delivering high-quality, patient-centered care. Here are three fundamental components that health care providers can focus on to cultivate and sustain compassionate care (Fig. 4.2).

### Leading with Purpose: The Power of Intentional Service in Health Care

Serving by intention is the foundation of compassionate care. It begins with a conscious decision to prioritize the well-being of patients in every interaction. This intentional approach requires health care providers to consistently focus on the patient's needs beyond just the physical symptoms they present. It involves an active commitment to see the person behind the illness, to understand their fears, hopes, and unique circumstances, and to respond with empathy and kindness.

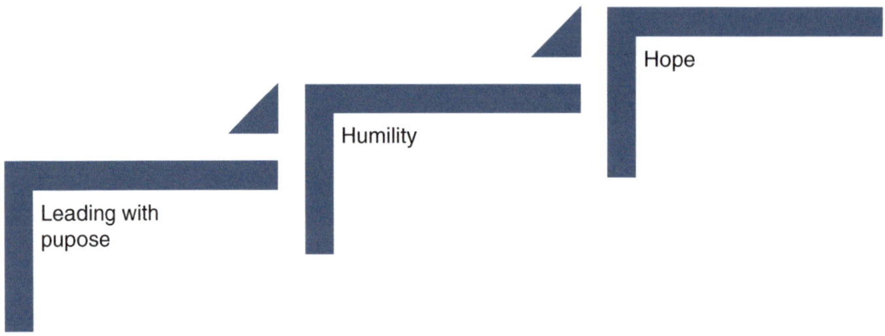


**Fig. 4.2** Steps to cultivating compassionate care

Intentional service means health care providers do not simply go through the motions of care but rather engage deeply with their patients. This engagement is characterized by active listening, where the provider gives full attention to the patient, seeking to understand their words and the emotions and concerns beneath them. This approach transforms routine clinical encounters into opportunities for genuine connection and healing.

In health care, the feelings patients carry with them long after their treatment has ended are often shaped by the compassion—or lack thereof—shown by their providers. By serving with intention, health care providers can ensure their patients feel valued, respected, and cared for, which can profoundly impact their overall experience and outcomes.

Additionally, serving by intention requires health care providers to remain present and mindful in each patient interaction. In a busy clinical setting, becoming distracted or viewing patients as just another item on a to-do list can be easy. However, intentional service calls for providers to slow down, even if only for a moment, to fully engage with each patient. This presence enhances the patient's experience and helps the provider feel more connected and fulfilled in their work.

Serving by intention is also closely aligned with "mindful medicine," where health care providers practice mindfulness to stay fully engaged and present during patient care. As Dr. Jon Kabat-Zinn, a pioneer in mindfulness-based stress reduction, explains, "Mindfulness means paying attention in a particular way: on purpose, in the present moment, and nonjudgmentally" [13]. This approach allows providers to be more attuned to their patients' needs and to respond with greater empathy and compassion.

Leading with purpose through intentional service in health care means showing up for patients not just as providers but as human beings who see beyond laboratory values and clinical algorithms. This became especially clear to me during a routine outpatient visit with a transplant recipient whose kidney function had begun to decline—several years after what had once been a life-restoring kidney transplant.

He came to the clinic that day for a follow-up after recent labs showed a steady rise in creatinine. The tone was different—quiet, withdrawn. As we sat together, I reviewed the numbers and outlined the next steps: potential biopsy, medication adjustments, and closer monitoring. But something in his body language—arms folded, eyes downcast—told me there was more going on than what the labs revealed.

So I paused. I set the medical record aside and asked, "How are you feeling about this?" That question opened the door.

He began to talk—first hesitantly, then more freely—about the mix of emotions they had been carrying. The gratitude they had felt after the transplant, how it had allowed them to rejoin life, reconnect with family, and even return to work. But now, the creeping rise in labs brought back all the old fears. "I feel like I'm losing the gift," he said. "Like I'm back at square one."

We talked about more than numbers that day. He shared the emotional exhaustion of living under constant surveillance by labs, the anxiety before every appointment, and the deep worry about what would happen next—whether he would need dialysis again or be around for his daughter's graduation.

Instead of rushing to fix it, I listened. I acknowledged the fear. Slowly, we reframed the path ahead—not in terms of loss but strength. We discussed how he could prepare emotionally, how to bring his family into the conversation, and how to focus on what still mattered deeply: relationships, purpose, and legacy.

By the end of the visit, something had shifted. There was still uncertainty, but now it was met with a sense of agency. "Thank you," he said quietly. "Today felt different. Like I wasn't just a patient—I was a person again."

That encounter reminded me that compassionate care in health care isn't just about offering answers—it's about offering presence. It's about honoring the whole narrative of a person's experience, even in a 30-min clinic visit. Sometimes, leading purposefully means stepping out of the medical script long enough to ask: "How are you doing?" And then staying long enough to hear the answer.

Let's turn to another powerful historical example of compassion in action—Clara Barton, founder of the American Red Cross. During the American Civil War, Barton emerged as a tireless advocate for wounded soldiers, earning the nickname "Angel of the Battlefield." Her story exemplifies what it means to serve with deep intention and compassion.

Barton began her work by collecting and distributing supplies for the Union Army. But soon, she realized the real need was not just on the home front, but on the battlefield itself. Defying social norms and significant bureaucratic resistance, she went directly to the front lines—often during active combat—to tend to the wounded. She brought with her not only medical supplies but also a calming presence, compassion, and a deep sense of duty.

In places like Antietam and Fredericksburg, Barton worked through the night, dressing wounds, comforting the dying, and organizing care with remarkable efficiency. She didn't merely treat injuries—she recognized the full humanity of the soldiers in front of her, often sitting beside them to offer words of comfort and assurance. One soldier later recalled, "She would kneel beside us, not as a nurse passing through, but as someone who truly saw us."

After the war, Barton took on another heart-wrenching task—helping families locate missing loved ones through the Office of Missing Soldiers. Driven by empathy and determination, she helped identify over 22,000 missing men. This work wasn't just administrative—it was deeply personal. Barton often wrote to grieving families herself, delivering both facts and comfort.

Her legacy culminated in the founding of the American Red Cross in 1881, expanding her compassionate mission globally. Barton once wrote, "You must never so much as think whether you like it or not, whether it is bearable or not; you must never think of anything except the need, and how to meet it." Her words and actions reflect the very core of intentional, compassionate service.

Clara Barton's legacy shows us true caregiving is not simply about treating illness or injury—it is about showing up fully, listening deeply, and responding with courage and heart. She reminds us the greatest impact we can have is not always in curing, but in caring.

Like the encounter with my transplant patient, her story illustrates health care providers' profound duty and privilege to serve with a heartfelt intention, acknowledging the entirety of a person's being. Through such stories, we see the timeless relevance of mindful and intentional care in fostering genuine connections, elevating the spirits of those served, and enriching the professional lives of those who serve.

## Humility

Humility is a cornerstone of compassionate care. In health care, humility involves recognizing that despite all the training, knowledge, and expertise one might possess, there is always more to learn and growth opportunities. Humility opens the door to continuous learning and improvement, as it encourages health care providers to remain curious, seek feedback, and be open to new perspectives.

The famous American writer and leadership guru John C. Maxwell defines humility as "an attitude where we understand who we are and appreciate and value other people" [22]. This attitude is essential in health care, where the power dynamics between provider and patient can sometimes lead to a sense of detachment or superiority. Humility breaks down these barriers, fostering a collaborative relationship where patients feel heard, respected, and involved in their care.

Humility in health care also means acknowledging the limitations of one's knowledge and abilities. No provider, no matter how skilled or experienced, can know everything or do everything perfectly. By embracing humility, providers can approach each patient interaction with a sense of openness and willingness to learn, whether from the patient, their family, or other health care team members.

Success in medicine is not just about curing diseases or performing procedures; it is about building trust, fostering collaboration, and creating an environment where patients feel safe and supported. Humility allows health care providers to admit when they do not have all the answers, ask for help when needed, and continually strive to improve their practice.

Humility also plays a critical role in building robust and effective health care teams. In a multidisciplinary environment, where doctors, nurses, technicians, and other professionals work together to care for patients, humility is the glue that holds the team together. It encourages mutual respect, open communication, and a willingness to learn from one another. This collaborative spirit is essential for delivering comprehensive, patient-centered care.

Moreover, humility extends beyond interactions with patients and colleagues to include a broader recognition of the complexity and unpredictability of health and illness. This perspective underscores the importance of seeing patients as whole persons with lives, stories, and experiences far beyond their medical conditions. By approaching each patient with humility, health care providers can offer genuinely compassionate and holistic care.

During my residency, in the heart of a busy intensive care unit, I first truly understood the power of humility in medicine. The ICU was where decisions often danced on the fine line between life and death—a relentless environment that demanded precision and confidence. As a resident, I felt the constant pressure to know, perform, and save. But it was there, between the sound of ventilators and beeping monitors, that I learned sometimes our greatest strength lies in admitting what we do not know.

One patient stands out vividly—a woman in her early 50s battling a rare and aggressive autoimmune disorder that had ravaged her organs. Her case was very complex. Despite being cared for by some of the brightest minds, her condition refused to follow the textbook. Each intervention seemed to buy her time, but none could turn the tide. I remember the night her oxygen levels plummeted despite everything we were doing. I stood by her bedside, reviewing every note, every lab, every imaging result. I felt the weight of expectation from my seniors and the family's hopeful eyes outside the room. I was supposed to know what to do. But I didn't. After exhausting every immediate option, I took a step back. Instead of pretending certainty, I chose honesty. I sat beside her, her breathing labored, but her gaze still steady. I explained we were doing everything we could, but her condition was proving to be more complex than we had anticipated. I admitted we didn't have a clear solution yet. Her eyes didn't fill with fear or anger as I had expected. Instead, they softened.

"Thank you for telling me the truth," she whispered. "I just need to know you're with me, even if you don't have all the answers." That conversation changed everything. She began sharing details about her body—how subtle shifts in her breathing pattern felt before these downturns, how certain positions eased her discomfort. These were insights no scan or test could reveal. With her input, we adjusted her positioning, tweaked her oxygen settings, and initiated small interventions that, while not curative, gave her some relief and dignity. But her disease was unrelenting. Despite our collective efforts, her condition deteriorated over the following days. One evening, surrounded by her family, she took her final breath.

I stood with her husband and daughter afterward, my chest tight with grief and a gnawing sense of inadequacy. I offered apologies for not being able to save her. But before I could finish, her husband placed a hand on my shoulder.

"You gave us more than medicine," he said. "You gave her respect. You listened. And you stayed with us until the end. That meant everything." In that moment, I understood humility in its purest form. It is not a weakness. It is the courage to be honest when the path is unclear, the strength to listen when answers elude us, and the grace to walk with patients and families—even to the end. That lesson stayed with me far beyond residency. The ICU machines and monitors taught me the science of healing. But it was that patient—and her family—who taught me its heart.

That encounter not only reshaped my understanding of medicine—it connected me to a lineage of healers who have practiced with deep humility and reverence for the human experience. One such figure was Dr. Paul Farmer. Dr. Paul Farmer co-founded Partners In Health (PIH), which provides high-quality health care in underserved areas. His approach to medicine was grounded in humility, understanding that every patient, no matter their economic situation or where they live, deserves respect and thorough care—one of the most memorable moments in his career occurred in Haiti's central plateau, where he dedicated himself to tackling the tuberculosis epidemic. Even with his education from some of the finest universities globally, Farmer frequently encountered medical challenges that no textbook could have prepared him for. He recognized the importance of complementing his academic knowledge with insights from the local community and their practices.

Farmer's humility truly shone through in blending modern medical treatments with community-focused health strategies. He didn't just tackle the diseases; he also considered the socio-economic issues, such as poverty and the lack of clean water, that affected health. His deep respect for local traditions and eagerness to learn from community members were vital to his achievements. For instance, when he worked with a young boy suffering from a multi-drug-resistant strain of tuberculosis, Farmer tailored his treatment plan after gaining insight into the boy's family circumstances and the herbal remedies they relied on. This holistic approach not only enhanced the boy's health but also fostered trust within the community, demonstrating Farmer truly valued their wisdom and input [8, 15].

Dr. Paul Farmer's journey illustrates humility in health care goes beyond recognizing one's limits; it's about embracing and learning from the communities we serve. This humility empowered him to develop more effective and respectful treatment strategies, significantly improving Haiti's patient outcomes and public health.

By admitting our vulnerabilities and embracing our limitations, we can build stronger connections with our patients and create a caring environment where true healing is fostered medically and emotionally. This humility transforms good physicians into great ones, allowing us to treat not just the disease but also the person living with it.

## Always Spread Hope

We'll talk about hope in more detail later in the book. Hope is a powerful and transformative force in health care. It is not merely an abstract concept but a vital component of compassionate care that can significantly influence patient experience and outcomes. Hope gives patients the strength to face their challenges, the resilience to endure complex treatments, and the motivation to engage actively in their recovery.

Creating an environment of hope begins with the health care provider's attitude and approach. Providers who convey a sense of optimism, even when dealing with uncertainty or adversity, can instill hope in their patients. This does not mean offering false hope or unrealistic expectations, but focusing on what is possible, what can be done, and how the patient can participate in their care to achieve the best possible outcome.

Spreading hope also involves helping patients find meaning and purpose in their experiences. This can be particularly important for patients facing long-term or terminal illnesses, where the focus may shift from cure to comfort, quality of life, and emotional and spiritual well-being. Providers can support patients in setting realistic goals, finding joy in small victories, and maintaining a sense of dignity and agency, even under challenging circumstances.

Moreover, hope is not just for patients; health care providers must also cultivate hope within themselves to sustain compassion and resilience. The demands of health care can be overwhelming, and without hope, providers are at risk of burnout and compassion fatigue. By maintaining a hopeful outlook, providers can find meaning and fulfillment in their work, even during daily challenges and stresses.

Viktor Frankl, a Holocaust survivor and psychiatrist, profoundly understood the importance of hope and meaning while facing suffering. In his book *Men's Search for Meaning*, he wrote, "When we are no longer able to change a situation, we are challenged to change ourselves" [9]. This insight is particularly relevant in health care, where providers often face situations beyond their control. Providers can navigate these challenges with compassion and grace by fostering hope and meaning for themselves and their patients.

In practical terms, spreading hope in health care might involve simple acts of kindness, such as a reassuring smile, a gentle touch, or words of encouragement. It could mean listening to a patient's fears and concerns, offering support during a difficult decision, or helping them see the positive aspects of their situation. While seemingly minor, these acts can profoundly impact a patient's outlook and experience.

Throughout my medical training, I realized providing hope is a crucial yet sometimes overlooked aspect of patient care. While accuracy and presenting patients with facts are important, it is equally essential to maintain a sense of hope. I learned that while honesty and data are necessary, they must be accompanied by hope. Patients find comfort in hope rather than statistics, as it fuels their resilience and guides them through challenging times.

This vital aspect of compassionate care came to life during my time with a patient facing a tough fight against a severe form of lymphoma following his kidney transplant. His diagnosis was challenging, and the journey ahead was filled with complexities and unknowns. Naturally, he approached his situation with a heavy heart; the burden of his illness dimmed the light of hope in his expression. Seeing his struggle, I understood how important it was for me to step in—not only as his doctor but also as a source of hope in the dark times of his battle. In our sessions, rather than just concentrating on the medical specifics and the overwhelming statistics, I highlighted the possibilities for joy and personal accomplishments, even in the face of his illness. We talked about more than just his treatment; we shared his love for gardening, his pride in his grandchildren's successes, and his hopes of watching them grow up.

One day, noticing his passion for gardening, I thought it would be nice to share some photos from my dad's garden that highlighted the stunning blooms across the seasons. I shared stories about my dad's passion for gardening, reminiscing about the times I saw him plant seeds, unsure of the outcome, yet watching them flourish despite the challenges—much like nurturing hope during difficult moments. Our conversations seemed to ignite a sense of hope in him, too; his face would light up as we linked the resilience of nature to his journey through treatment. As the weeks turned into months, his condition improved enough for him to be discharged with ongoing outpatient support. On the day he left, he gave me a small packet of flower seeds—a lovely gesture representing the hope we had cultivated together. He shared his wish to plant these seeds as a symbol of his continued recovery and the optimism for the future we built during our sessions.

This personal experience highlights the incredible power of hope in health care. By emphasizing his strengths and passions, I helped him rediscover the resilience and motivation to continue battling his illness. It reminded me once again that while we may not always find a cure, we can always choose to bring light and hope into our patients' lives, guiding them through their most challenging moments with strength and dignity. Through acts of kindness and understanding, we not only address the illness but also connect with the human spirit, which is truly at the heart of healing.

In conclusion, cultivating compassionate care is an ongoing journey that requires health care providers to serve with intention, practice humility, and always spread hope. These principles are theoretical ideals and practical approaches that can transform how care is delivered and experienced. By embracing these components, health care providers can ensure their care is clinically effective, deeply human, and compassionate.

## Compassionate Care in End-of-Life Situations

Offering compassionate care during the end-of-life stage is both a rewarding and emotionally challenging part of medical practice. It requires health care providers to embody deep empathy, respect, and sensitivity as they address the clinical aspects of care and the emotional and spiritual needs of patients and their families.

In his deeply insightful book, *The Best Care Possible*, Dr. Ira Byock, a physician, author, and keynote speaker, advocates for a palliative care approach that transcends merely alleviating physical symptoms. He urges health care providers to recognize that the burdens faced at the end of life are often far more complex, extending beyond pain management to profound emotional and existential challenges. Patients nearing the end of their journey frequently grapple with grief over impending loss, fear of the unknown, and the weight of unfulfilled hopes or fractured relationships.

Byock emphasizes that truly compassionate care requires addressing these human dimensions with the same urgency as clinical concerns. He reminds us that patients are not defined solely by their diagnoses; they are individuals with rich, unique life stories, personal values, and aspirations that remain deeply significant even as their bodies decline. Their sense of dignity and wholeness can be preserved when caregivers acknowledge their humanity—offering not only medical expertise but also empathy, respect, and the space to find closure and meaning. Byock's work challenges us to rethink end-of-life care, urging us to ensure that patients do not simply die free of pain but also live their final days with purpose, peace, and the knowledge that they matter [3].

During my residency, I had the privilege of learning from Dr. Michelle Reisner, a remarkable geriatric and palliative care physician whose approach to caring for terminally ill patients left a lasting imprint on my journey as a doctor. Her ability to be present with patients in the final moments of their lives was nothing short of extraordinary. Dr. Reisner demonstrated that providing comfort at the end of life was not merely about controlling pain or managing symptoms—it was about honoring the person before us, embracing their fears, and affirming their dignity when time was slipping away. I vividly remember the first time I accompanied her to the bedside of a patient who was taking her final breaths. There was no rush, no clinical urgency—only a profound stillness as she leaned in gently, speaking softly to the patient, holding her hand. She asked about her life, her family, and her happiest memories. She truly listened, allowing her stories to fill the room, even when her voice trembled or weakened. She reminded me that, in those final minutes, patients do not ask about laboratory results or medical breakthroughs; they speak of love, regrets, and those they will leave behind.

One experience particularly stands out. I watched as Dr. Reisner sat with an older woman whose life was drawing to a close. The woman's breathing was shallow, but her eyes flickered with recognition as Dr. Reisner spoke her name and reassured her that she was not alone. She encouraged the patient to talk if she wished but reassured her silence was also welcome. The woman chose to talk—she spoke of her late husband, their garden in springtime, and the laughter of her grandchildren. Dr. Reisner held her hand the entire time, occasionally offering simple, heartfelt words: "*That sounds beautiful… He must have loved you dearly… You gave them so much.*"

I realized that day that comfort in dying is not just about morphine or oxygen; it is about being seen and heard—being reminded your life matters. In those moments, I learned the power of simply *being there*. A hand on a shoulder, a gentle nod, a shared tear—these gestures transcend medicine. They tell the patient, *You are not alone. You are valued. Your story matters.* Dr. Reisner taught me that the final chapter of a patient's life deserves as much attention and reverence as its beginning. Her work taught me that being a physician is not just about saving lives but also about walking with patients—even to the very end—with grace, humility, and unwavering compassion.

In his groundbreaking book, *Being Mortal*, Dr. Atul Gawande, surgeon, writer, and public health researcher, offers a profoundly human perspective on aging, illness, and the often overlooked importance of quality of life in the face of mortality.

Gawande challenges the conventional mindset within the health care system, which is frequently driven by a relentless pursuit of prolonging life—sometimes at the cost of the patient's dignity, comfort, and personal values. He argues this singular focus on survival can lead to aggressive interventions that extend days but diminish their meaning. Through poignant patient stories and reflections on his family's experiences, Gawande highlights the unintended harm that can arise when medicine views death solely as the ultimate enemy to defeat. Instead, he calls for a paradigm shift—one that centers on what truly matters to patients as they approach the end of their lives. He emphasizes that the goal of care should not always be to extend life at all costs, but to ensure the time patients have left is filled with meaning, autonomy, and comfort.

Gawande advocates for open, honest conversations between doctors and patients—discussions that explore what patients value most when time is limited. For some, it may be the ability to stay home surrounded by family. For others, it might be maintaining independence for as long as possible or simply enjoying a favorite meal. This patient-centered approach reframes life's final chapter, transforming it from a battleground of medical interventions into a period where patients can live on their terms. Gawande's philosophy underscores that while medicine's advances have given us the power to extend life, its true purpose lies in enhancing the quality of the life we are preserving—right until the very end. His work serves as a powerful reminder that, ultimately, a "good death" is not about defeating death but about enabling patients to face it with dignity, peace, and a sense of completion [10].

In his profoundly moving memoir, *When Breath Becomes Air*, Dr. Paul Kalanithi, writer and neurosurgeon, takes readers on a deeply personal journey from being a brilliant neurosurgeon at the peak of his career to becoming a terminal lung cancer patient grappling with his mortality. His transition from healer to patient unveils a raw, unfiltered view of what it means to confront death—not as a distant reality for others but as an imminent certainty for oneself.

Kalanithi's reflections reveal the limitations of modern medicine in matters of the soul. He challenges the medical community's tendency to focus solely on prolonging life, reminding us that when a cure is no longer possible, what matters most is ensuring a patient's remaining days are filled with meaning, dignity, and human connection. Throughout his illness, Kalanithi came to understand that patients facing the end of life are often left navigating an emotional and spiritual wilderness. The clinical discussions about prognosis and treatment options, though necessary, frequently overlook the person behind the disease—their fears, their hopes, and their desire to retain a sense of self as their body weakens. He emphasizes that the role of a physician, especially when death approaches, is not simply to delay the inevitable but to guide patients through this challenging passage with compassion, honesty, and respect. In these final stages, compassionate care becomes the most powerful form of healing.

Kalanithi describes how the simple yet profound acts of listening, holding a hand, acknowledging suffering, and honoring what matters most to the patient can provide comfort far beyond any medical intervention. He writes about how his medical providers, who treated him with humanity—who saw him not just as a cancer patient but as a husband, a soon-to-be father, and a man longing to live meaningfully—helped him face his mortality with a sense of peace and acceptance. His story is a reminder that while medicine can extend life, it cannot always restore it to what it once was. When death is near, the medical provider's role evolves—from fighting disease to ensuring patients can live fully in their final days, however few they may be. Through compassion—being present, listening without judgment, and affirming the patient's dignity—we offer the greatest gift: the chance for a "good death," in which the patient is not merely defined by their illness but is seen, valued, and allowed to shape their final moments in a way that reflects the life they have lived.

Kalanithi's legacy endures as a call to all health care providers, urging us to recognize our duty extends beyond medicine in the face of death. It demands we bring our humanity to the bedside, standing alongside patients as they face life's final transition, ensuring they are not alone and their last chapter is written with grace, comfort, and dignity [14].

These philosophies come to life in many wonderful ways: holding a patient's hand, encouraging family visits, sharing music or personal interests, and engaging in heartfelt conversations. While these actions may seem simple, they have a tremendous impact. They offer comfort to patients, reminding them they are not alone and are cherished and loved.

Additionally, compassionate care also means being there for families facing the emotional challenges of impending loss. This support includes providing regular updates to keep them informed, involving them in care decisions, and offering guidance on coping with grief. Health care providers play a vital role in connecting patients with their families, ensuring everyone feels prepared and supported during this difficult time.

In sum, compassionate end-of-life care is not just about managing physical symptoms but about honoring the person, recognizing their life's worth, and supporting their family through the transition. This comprehensive approach not only enhances patient outcomes but also ensures the end of life is as prosperous and dignified as its beginning, profoundly impacting all involved.

## Compassionate Care Through the Lens of Generational Understanding

Health care providers must appreciate the value of being sensitive to the various generations when building meaningful patient relationships. By understanding the distinct preferences, communication styles, and health beliefs of each generation—from the Silent Generation to the Zoomers—health care providers can show professional respect and significantly enhance patient satisfaction and health results [1]. Let's briefly examine the different generations and how medical professionals can tailor their approach to each one. Compassionate care through the lens of generational understanding is summarized in Table 4.1.

**Table 4.1** Understanding care through the lens of generational understanding

| Generation | Birth years | Defining characteristics | Preferred communication style | Health care approach |
|---|---|---|---|---|
| Silent generation | 1928–1945 | Cautious, resilient, values tradition, respect for authority, disciplined work ethic | Formal, face-to-face, written letters prefer being addressed by titles | Prefers thorough explanations in simple terms, values respect and patience, and appreciates providers who take time and maintain a professional demeanor |
| Baby boomers | 1946–1964 | Strong work ethic, independent, driven by success, shaped by social movements, values, purpose | Direct, face-to-face, values personal touch, open to technology like email | Desires active participation in health care decisions, values transparency, expects detailed explanations, and prefers collaboration with health care providers |
| Generation X | 1965–1980 | Independent, adaptable, skeptical of authority, practical, resourceful | Direct, efficient, prefer honesty over formality, comfortable with tech | Appreciates evidence-based information, values efficiency, prefers digital convenience and personalized care, and expects respect for their research and decision-making involvement |
| Millennials | 1981–1996 | Tech-savvy, collaborative, socially conscious, values work-life balance and well-being | Digital communication (email, text, online portals) values quick responses | Prefers convenience-driven solutions (telehealth, online scheduling), values transparency and shared decision-making, and expects providers to respect their knowledge and digital research |
| Generation Z | 1997–2010 | Tech-native, values individuality, diversity, and social justice, entrepreneurial, independent | Quick, visual, digital-first (messaging apps, social media), values immediacy | Expects digital access to health care services (apps, telehealth), values authenticity and transparency, and appreciates providers who align with their values of inclusivity and social responsibility |

## Silent Generation

The Silent Generation, born between 1928 and 1945, was shaped by significant historical events such as the Great Depression, World War II, and the early years of the Cold War. These experiences fostered a sense of caution, resilience, and adherence to tradition within the generation. Many members of this group grew up in economic instability and political tension, cultivating a strong work ethic and a deep respect for authority. They are often characterized by their quiet perseverance and disciplined approach to life, placing high value on duty and responsibility.

In terms of communication, the Silent Generation prefers more formal, direct methods. They value in-person, face-to-face conversations and are accustomed to the formality of written letters. While many have adapted to newer forms of communication, such as email or even text messaging, their preference often remains with traditional, slower-paced interactions. They associate formality with respect and find comfort in well-structured, personal exchanges. For instance, they are likely to appreciate being addressed by formal titles, such as "Mr" or "Mrs," as it aligns with their values of decorum and professionalism.

Engaging effectively with this generation requires a thoughtful and respectful approach for health care providers. Taking the time to establish a rapport through direct, polite communication is crucial. They may appreciate thorough explanations of medical information delivered in simple, easy-to-understand terms. Given their cautious nature, they may require more time to process information and make decisions about their health, and it is essential to allow for this without rushing them. Respect for their values, combined with a measured, authoritative demeanor, can foster trust, ensuring health care providers can communicate effectively and provide optimal care to members of the Silent Generation.

## Baby Boomers

The Baby Boomer generation, born between 1946 and 1964, experienced a period marked by post-war economic prosperity and significant social and cultural shifts. Many Baby Boomers grew up witnessing movements for civil rights, gender equality, and political reform, contributing to their openness to change and innovation. This generation is often recognized for its strong work ethic, independence, and desire for self-fulfillment. The values of hard work and success were instilled early in their lives, leading many Boomers to define themselves through their careers and personal achievements. As they age, they seek purpose and engagement in their professional and personal lives.

With communication, Baby Boomers prefer precise, direct interactions. Unlike previous generations, they are more comfortable expressing their thoughts and engaging in meaningful discussions. They appreciate opportunities to ask questions and contribute to conversations, particularly regarding decisions about their health or personal matters. While they are familiar with technology, such as email and smartphones, and regularly use digital methods of communication, they still value the personal touch of face-to-face interactions. Personal communication helps reinforce trust and understanding, which is essential for this generation, especially in complex decision-making scenarios.

For health care providers, it is essential to recognize the Baby Boomers' desire for active participation in their health care decisions. This generation values transparency, detailed explanations, and various options for them to consider. Collaboration is critical to building a trusting relationship. By involving them in the decision-making process, respecting their knowledge and life experience, and providing them with all necessary information, health care professionals can better meet their needs. In turn, this collaborative approach helps Baby Boomers feel more in control of their health and fosters a stronger and more engaged doctor-patient relationship.

## Generation X

Generation X, born between 1965 and 1980, grew up during a transformative time marked by rapid technological advancements and significant economic shifts. They witnessed the transition from analog to digital media, the rise of personal computers, and the early stages of the internet, all contributing to their adaptability and independence. Many Gen Xers grew up in dual-income or single-parent households, leading them to develop a strong sense of self-reliance and resourcefulness from an early age. Their formative years were also shaped by major economic events, such as the oil crisis of the 1970s and the economic boom of the 1980s, providing them with firsthand experience of both prosperity and financial instability. This mix of experiences has fostered a practical, no-nonsense approach to problem-solving, evident in their professional and personal lives.

Known for their skeptical nature, Gen X tends to question authority and traditional systems, a mindset shaped by events like the Watergate scandal and the shifting political landscape of the late twentieth century. This skepticism extends to how they consume information and interact with the world. They appreciate efficiency and direct communication, valuing honesty and straightforwardness over formality. Growing up in the pre-digital and digital eras, they are comfortable navigating in-person interactions and digital communications. They are adept at using technology for practical purposes, such as managing their finances or health records. Yet, they also appreciate the personal touch of face-to-face engagement when necessary.

For health care providers, meeting the needs of Generation X patients requires a balance of modern convenience and personalized care. Gen Xers are likely to come prepared with their research, as they seek out information independently before making decisions. Health care providers should be ready to offer evidence-based explanations and respect their desire to be informed participants in their health care journey. Gen X values the integration of technology, such as online health portals for appointment scheduling and access to medical records. Still, they also appreciate providers who take the time to engage with them. Combining the benefits of modern technology with attentive, personalized care can help establish trust and create a cooperative, well-informed health care experience for this tech-savvy yet independent generation.

## Millennials

Born between 1981 and 1996, millennials are the first generation to have grown up with technology at their fingertips, shaping their values and expectations in many aspects of life, including health care. They have experienced the rapid rise of the internet, smartphones, and social media, which has ingrained in them a preference for instant access to information and services. This generation values a healthy work-life balance, often prioritizing flexibility and well-being over traditional workplace structures. In addition, millennials tend to be more socially conscious than previous generations, placing importance on environmental sustainability, equality, and corporate social responsibility in their decision-making processes. This also carries over into their health care expectations, where they seek providers who reflect similar values and practices.

Millennials are known for their collaborative nature and positive outlook on life. They seek experiences where their opinions are valued and expect transparency from organizations they interact with, including those in health care. Convenience is vital for this generation, and they expect health care services to fit seamlessly into their busy lives. They prefer digital communication channels like email, text messaging, and online patient portals, allowing them to manage appointments and prescriptions and access their health records on the go. Researching and accessing medical information electronically empowers them to be proactive in their health care decisions, often arriving at appointments with extensive background knowledge of their conditions and treatment options. Speed and efficiency are highly valued, as they expect quick responses and results from their health care providers.

For health care providers, effectively engaging with millennials requires combining technology driven solutions and personal engagement. Offering online appointment scheduling, telemedicine options, and easy access to medical records through patient portals is essential for meeting their expectations of convenience. However, personal engagement remains crucial for fostering a lasting provider-patient relationship. Millennials appreciate health care providers who respect their informed perspectives and involve them in decision-making. By offering transparent communication, providing clear treatment options, and addressing their questions directly, health care providers can build trust and encourage collaboration with their Millennial patients. This balance of modern digital solutions and personalized care helps millennials feel empowered, respected, and actively involved in managing their health.

## Generation Z

Generation Z, typically recognized as those born from 1997 to 2010, is the most internet-fluent and tech-savvy generation, having grown up in a world where smartphones, social media, and advanced technology were already prevalent. From a young age, they have been exposed to digital platforms that allow instant access to information and the ability to communicate globally, which has profoundly influenced their worldview and expectations. Gen Z places a high value on individuality, diversity, and inclusivity, prizing environments where differences are celebrated and personal expression is encouraged. Their pragmatic and entrepreneurial outlook has been shaped by growing up during global unrest, economic instability, and rapid technological advancement, prompting them to be more independent and self-reliant.

In terms of communication, Generation Z favors quick, efficient, and often visual methods, such as messaging apps, short-form video content, and social media platforms like Instagram, TikTok, and Snapchat. They expect on-demand access to information and are used to multitasking across multiple digital channels. This generation is less likely to rely on traditional means of communication, such as phone calls or emails, preferring the immediacy of direct messaging or online chat systems. Their comfort with technology extends to how they approach their health care needs, where they expect easy access to services such as online appointment scheduling, telehealth consultations, and digital health records. This aligns with their preference for self-service options that allow them to take control of their health care journey without unnecessary delays.

A tech-forward, innovative approach is crucial for health care providers to effectively engage with Generation Z. Offering digital platforms that integrate seamlessly with their daily routines, such as mobile apps for appointment scheduling and health tracking, is likely to resonate with this generation. Moreover, Gen Z values authenticity and transparency in all interactions, so health care providers should ensure their communication is straightforward, clear, and genuine. Additionally, this generation is highly conscious of social justice issues, and they expect the brands and services they interact with, including health care, to reflect their values of inclusivity and social responsibility. Providers who embrace diversity, practice environmental sustainability, and maintain an active presence in social causes will likely build stronger connections with Generation Z patients, ensuring they feel heard, respected, and empowered in managing their health.

In conclusion, grasping the distinctions between generations is more than just interacting with patients—it's a heartfelt journey toward delivering compassionate care. By appreciating each generation's unique communication styles, beliefs, and expectations, health care professionals can transcend traditional medical boundaries. Medical providers go beyond merely treating ailments; they nurture individuals, each with their own unique stories and backgrounds that influence their health and wellness perspectives. As medical providers enhance their understanding of generational sensitivity, they can foster a health care system that is practical, profoundly empathetic, and attuned to the human experience. Let's keep listening, learning, and connecting across all ages because it's within the beautiful blend of generational voices that we can discover true healing harmony.

In the diverse world of my medical practice, I've encountered distinct differences in generational expectations, primarily through my experiences with two unforgettable patients: Mrs. A from the Silent Generation and Mrs. B, who represents the Millennial generation.

Mrs. A, born during the tremulous 1940s, carried the weight of her era with dignified grace permeating her approach to health care. Each visit, she arrived with her questions meticulously noted in a worn, leather-bound journal, her elegant handwriting filling the pages. Her questions were not just inquiries but reflections of a lifetime lived within the rigid frameworks of respect and formality. For Mrs. A, medical appointments were profound engagements deserving of time and thoughtful deliberation. She valued comprehensive dialogues and expected her voice to be heard clearly, reflecting her generational values of structure and detailed understanding.

Then there was Mrs. B, a true Millennial who moved to a different beat. Growing up in the digital age of the late 1980s, her approach to health care matched the quick pace of the technology that shaped her life. She preferred digital communication—emails, texts, and health apps were her go-to tools. She arrived at appointments well-prepared, equipped with research from the internet, and eager to discuss, debate, and analyze treatment options with a focus on efficiency. Her questions were sharp and to the point, often challenging traditional medical practices with the confidence that comes from having easy access to information.

The juxtaposition of these encounters came to a head one crisp autumn morning. Mrs. A had just left my office, leaving behind the scent of her floral perfume and a room still echoing with our conversation's thorough, deliberate pace. Then Mrs. B breezed in, smartphone in hand, a stark contrast with her quick, clipped speech and a gaze that seldom wavered from the screen of her device.

In those moments, the differences between Mrs. A's careful, traditional engagement and Mrs. B's brisk, tech-driven interactions painted a vivid picture of the generational divide. With Mrs. A, the challenge was to weave her narrative into her medical care, respecting her need for depth and reflection. With Mrs. B, it was about keeping pace with her rapid-fire questions and integrating the latest digital tools to provide immediate, evidence-based responses.

These experiences go beyond simple medical consultations; they are vibrant, engaging interactions that challenge a health care provider's ability to communicate effectively, which is the cornerstone of compassionate care. They underscore the importance of adjusting to diverse expectations, making sure every patient feels appreciated and understood, no matter their age or background. By connecting across generational divides, I honor the unique needs of my patients and create a rich tapestry of care that respects the past while looking forward to the future, beautifully illustrating the evolution of patient care through the years.

## Teaching Compassion in Medical Education

Despite its critical role in patient care, compassion has historically been underemphasized in medical education. The rigorous demands of medical training often focus heavily on clinical skills, technical knowledge, and the science of medicine, sometimes at the expense of the art of healing. However, there is a growing recognition within the medical community that compassion is not just an optional quality for health care providers but a core component of effective medical practice.

Incorporating compassion into medical education requires a fundamental shift in both curriculum and culture. Medical schools and training programs must go beyond teaching the mechanics of medicine and prioritize the development of compassionate communication skills, emotional intelligence, and ethical decision-making. This holistic approach to medical education recognizes that while clinical knowledge is essential, the ability to connect with patients on a human level is equally important for delivering high-quality care.

One effective method for teaching compassion in medical education is structured reflective practice. Reflective practice involves encouraging medical students and trainees to reflect on their experiences, emotions, and patient interactions. This process helps students develop a deeper understanding of the human side of medicine, fostering empathy and compassion. Reflective practice can take many forms, including journaling, group discussions, and debriefing sessions after clinical encounters. By reflecting on their experiences, students can identify moments where compassion made a difference and opportunities where more compassionate care could have been provided.

The value of reflective practice is underscored by the words of the renowned educator and philosopher John Dewey, who stated, "We do not learn from experience… we learn from reflecting on experience" [6]. In medical education, this reflection helps students internalize the lessons of compassionate care and apply them in future patient interactions. It encourages them to consider the emotional and psychological aspects of patient care, often as important as the physical aspects.

Role-playing exercises are another powerful tool for teaching compassion in medical education. These exercises allow students to practice compassionate communication in a controlled environment, where they can receive feedback from instructors and peers. By simulating difficult conversations—such as delivering bad news, discussing end-of-life care, or addressing patient fears—students can develop the skills to navigate these situations with empathy and sensitivity. Role-playing also helps students build confidence in their ability to handle emotionally charged interactions, which are common in medical practice.

In addition to classroom instruction and role-playing, real-world clinical experiences are crucial for developing compassion in medical students. These experiences allow students to observe and learn from experienced health care providers who model compassionate care. Mentorship is vital in this context. When students see their mentors demonstrating compassion in their interactions with patients, they are more likely to emulate those behaviors. As the saying goes, "Compassion is caught, not taught." By witnessing compassion in action, students can appreciate its impact on patient care and understand its integral role in medicine.

Moreover, fostering a culture of compassion within medical institutions is essential for reinforcing these lessons. Medical schools and hospitals must create environments where compassion is valued and encouraged at all levels. This includes supporting health care providers struggling with burnout or compassion fatigue and recognizing and rewarding acts of kindness. By embedding compassion into the institutional culture, medical educators can ensure it becomes a natural part of the care students and providers offer their patients.

As Dr. Rachel Naomi Remen, a pioneer in integrative medicine, wisely observed, "The most critical part of the curriculum is the invisible curriculum, the one that students learn by observing the lives of their teachers" [25]. This invisible curriculum includes the attitudes, behaviors, and values students absorb through interactions with faculty, staff, and peers. Those in leadership positions visibly prioritize compassion, and it sends a powerful message to students about the kind of health care provider they should aspire to be.

Incorporating compassion into medical education also helps students build the resilience they will need to navigate the emotional challenges of their careers. Medicine is a demanding field, and health care providers are frequently exposed to suffering, loss, and high-stress situations. Compassionate care not only benefits patients but also supports the well-being of health care providers. By learning to approach their work with compassion, students can develop a more profound sense of purpose and fulfillment, which can sustain them through the inevitable challenges they will face in their careers.

In short, teaching compassion in medical education is essential for preparing future health care providers to deliver holistic, patient-centered care. This requires a shift in curriculum and culture, emphasizing reflective practice, role-playing exercises, real-world clinical experiences, and mentorship. By prioritizing compassion alongside clinical skills, medical educators can ensure their students are equipped to treat diseases and care for the whole person. In medicine, this purpose is fulfilled when compassionate care becomes the cornerstone of practice, guiding every interaction between health care providers and their patients.

## Conclusion: Compassion as the Heart of Health Care

Compassionate care is not just a desirable quality but essential for achieving better patient clinical outcomes and preventing physician burnout. As Dr. Paul Kalanithi wrote in *When Breath Becomes Air*, "The physician's duty is not just to avoid death but to improve the quality of life, which means active and compassionate management of pain and suffering" [14]. Compassionate care allows health care providers to fulfill this duty, offering their patients medical treatment, emotional support, and hope.

We must integrate compassionate care into the curriculum of our future medical providers. By doing so, we can ensure the next generation of health care professionals is equipped with the technical skills to treat disease and the compassion to care for their patients honestly. Compassionate care allows health care providers to do just that—to find themselves in the service of those who need them most.

Compassion is the heart of health care. It transforms the act of providing medical care into a healing experience. It makes the difference between a patient feeling like a number and a patient feeling like a person. As we continue to advance in medicine and technology, let us not forget the timeless value of compassion—the essence of what it means to care.

**Take-Home Points**

- Compassion Enhances Patient Outcomes and Reduces Burnout.
- Connection Beyond Treatment Is Healing.
- Hope Is a Vital Part of Compassionate Care.
- Humility Strengthens the Doctor-Patient Relationship.
- Compassion Is an Active Practice, Not Just Emotion.

## References


1. Aziz F. Compassionate care through the lens of generational understanding. WMJ. 2024;123(2):68–9. https://www.ncbi.nlm.nih.gov/pubmed/38718227
2. Bus collision kills 6, injures nearly 50 in Sweden. 2007. https://www.chron.com/news/nation-world/article/Bus-collision-kills-6-injures-nearly-50-in-Sweden-1533717.php
3. Byock I. The best care possible: a physician's quest to transform care through the end of life. New York: Avery; 2012.
4. Chadwick MWN. Hippocratic writings. New York: Penguin Classics; 1984.
5. Debets MPM, Jansen I, Diepeveen M, Bogerd R, Molewijk BAC, Widdershoven GAM, Lombarts K. Compassionate care through the eyes of patients and physicians: an interview study. PLoS One. 2024;19(7):e0305007. https://doi.org/10.1371/journal.pone.0305007.
6. Dewey J. How we think: a restatement of the relation of reflective thinking to the educative process. Boston: DC Heath and Company; 1993.
7. Doohan I, Saveman BI. Need for compassion in prehospital and emergency care: a qualitative study on bus crash survivors' experiences. Int Emerg Nurs. 2015;23(2):115–9. https://doi.org/10.1016/j.ienj.2014.08.008.
8. Farmer P. Pathologies of power: health, human rights, and the new war on the poor. Berkeley: University of California Press; 2003.
9. Frankl VE. Man's search for meaning. Boston: Beacon Press; 1959.
10. Gawande A. Being mortal: medicine and what matters in the end. New York: Metropolitan Books; 2014.
11. Hojat M, Louis DZ, Markham FW, Wender R, Rabinowitz C, Gonnella JS. Physicians' empathy and clinical outcomes for diabetic patients. Acad Med. 2011;86(3):359–64. https://doi.org/10.1097/ACM.0b013e3182086fe1.
12. Howick J, Moscrop A, Mebius A, Fanshawe TR, Lewith G, Bishop FL, Mistiaen P, Roberts NW, Dieninyte E, Hu XY, Aveyard P, Onakpoya IJ. Effects of empathic and positive communication in health care consultations: a systematic review and meta-analysis. J R Soc Med. 2018;111(7):240–52. https://doi.org/10.1177/0141076818769477.
13. Kabat-Zinn J. Wherever you go, there you are: mindfulness meditation in everyday life. New York: Hyperion; 1984.
14. Kalanithi P. When breath becomes air. New York: Random House; 2016.

15. Kidder T. Mountains beyond mountains: the quest of Dr Paul Farmer, a man who would cure the world. New York: Random House Trade Paperbacks; 2003.
16. Lama D. The art of happiness. New York: Riverhead Books; 2009.
17. Lee Y, Seomun G. Compassion competence in nurses. ANS Adv Nurs Sci. 2016a;39(2):E54–66. https://doi.org/10.1097/ANS.0000000000000111.
18. Lee Y, Seomun G. Role of compassion competence among clinical nurses in professional quality of life. Int Nurs Rev. 2016b;63(3):381–7. https://doi.org/10.1111/inr.12295.
19. Levinson W, Roter DL, Mullooly JP, Dull VT, Frankel RM. Physician-patient communication. The relationship with malpractice claims among primary care physicians and surgeons. JAMA. 1997;277(7):553–9. https://doi.org/10.1001/jama.277.7.553.
20. Malenfant S, Jaggi P, Hayden KA, Sinclair S. Compassion in health care: an updated scoping review of the literature. BMC Palliat Care. 2022;21(1):80. https://doi.org/10.1186/s12904-022-00942-3.
21. Mandela N. Long walk to freedom: the autobiography of Nelson Mandela. New York: Little, Brown and Company; 1994.
22. Maxwell J. The 21 indispensable qualities of a leader: becoming the person others will want to follow. Nashville: Thomas Nelson; 1999.
23. Naisbitt J. High tech/high touch: technology and our search for meaning. New York: Broadway Books; 1999.
24. Peabody F. The Care of the Patient. JAMA. 1927;88:877–82.
25. Remen RN. Kitchen table wisdom: stories that heal. New York: Riverhead Books; 1996.
26. Rodriguez-Perez ME, Sandoval-Olvera F, Hernandez-Salinas H. Jean Dominique Larrey y su reconocimiento en Mexico [Jean Dominique Larrey and his recognition in Mexico]. Cir Cir. 2020;88(3):389–94. https://doi.org/10.24875/CIRU.19000870.
27. Shadyac T. Patch Adams. Universal Pictures; 1998.
28. Trzeciak S, Mazzarelli A. Compassionomics: the revolutionary scientific evidence that caring makes a difference. Pensacola: Studer Group; 2019.
29. Trzeciak S, Mazzarelli A. Wonder drug: 7 scientifically proven ways that serving others is the best medicine for yourself. New York: St. Martin's Press; 2022.

# 5 Communication

The sterile smell of disinfectant filled the air as Mr. Thompson sat in the corner of the exam room, his gaze fixed on the scuffed linoleum floor. His fingers tapped restlessly on his knee, betraying the turmoil within. At 58 years old, Mr. Thompson had spent his life as a devoted schoolteacher, guiding students with patience and care. But today, he felt powerless.

An hour earlier, he had received the news—stage II colorectal cancer. The words still echoed in his head, each syllable reverberating like a drumbeat.

*Cancer… Me? How could this happen? What now?*

He had barely heard the nurse's instructions afterward, feeling like the walls were closing in around him. His mind jumped to the worst—images of chemotherapy, weight loss, and his wife, Margaret, caring for him when she should be enjoying their retirement together.

Mr. Thompson didn't look up when Dr. Sarah Jennings entered the room with a clipboard. His shoulders were slumped, his breath shallow. "Mr Thompson?" Dr. Jennings greeted softly. "I'm Dr Jennings. I know this has been a tough morning."

Mr. Thompson gave a half-hearted nod but didn't meet her eyes.

Sensing his distress, Dr. Jennings set her clipboard aside and pulled a chair closer, so they were at eye level. She didn't immediately jump into medical details. Instead, she paused—giving Mr. Thompson the space to speak first. "Would you like to talk about what's on your mind?" she asked gently.

Mr. Thompson's voice was strained. "I don't even know where to start." He paused, his fingers clenching the edge of the examination table. "I… I just feel like everything's crashing down. No one explained what was going to happen. I don't know what I'm supposed to do next. Am I just supposed to sit and wait for bad news?"

The frustration in his voice was sharp, but Dr. Jennings didn't flinch. Instead, she nodded—a small gesture that acknowledged his pain. "I hear you," she said quietly.


F. Aziz, *The Healing Art of Connecting with Patients*,
https://doi.org/10.1007/978-3-032-03624-7_5

"This is overwhelming, and feeling like you're in the dark makes it even harder. Tell me what's worrying you most right now."

For a moment, Mr. Thompson hesitated, but then his words spilled like water from a broken dam. "I'm scared about what this means for Margaret… she's been through so much with her health. And my daughter is about to have her first baby. What if I'm not here to see my grandson grow up?" His voice cracked. "And what if I'm just too weak to keep going?"

He wiped his eyes roughly with the back of his hand. "I just don't know how to handle all this."

Dr. Jennings leaned in slightly, her posture calm but attentive. She let the silence linger momentarily—a crucial pause that settled Mr. Thompson's emotions. "I can't imagine how hard this must be," she said softly. "And you have every right to feel this way." She paused again, giving weight to her words. "But I want you to know—you're not alone in this."

For the first time, Mr. Thompson looked up.

"We have a dedicated team, specialists in oncology, surgeons, and people trained to support you emotionally and physically," she continued. "And I'll be with you through every step. We're not going to leave you guessing. We're going to make a plan—together."

Mr. Thompson's breathing slowed slightly. "A plan?" he repeated.

"Yes," Dr. Jennings said with a gentle smile. "Let's break this down. We'll start with your imaging results so we know exactly what we're dealing with. Then, I'll walk you through your treatment options. I'll be honest. There will be some challenges ahead, but you have options. And we'll tackle each decision one step at a time."

She reached for her notepad and began sketching a simple outline with clear, step-by-step points focused on action, not just medical jargon. Mr. Thompson's eyes followed her pen closely.

"And if at any point you feel overwhelmed or unsure," she added, "you can call me directly. We'll schedule regular check-ins so I can answer your questions."

Mr. Thompson let out a shaky breath. "You're saying… you'll be there?"

"Every step," Dr. Jennings affirmed.

For the first time that morning, Mr. Thompson's expression softened. The fear in his eyes had not disappeared, but it had shifted—replaced by something closer to hope.

"Thank you," he said quietly. "I feel like I can breathe again."

As Dr. Jennings walked him to the door, Mr. Thompson turned back. "I'm glad you took the time to listen," he said. "I don't feel so… lost anymore."

In this hypothetical scenario, Dr. Jennings effectively communicated with Mr. Thompson by practicing active listening, showing genuine empathy, and offering clear guidance. This interaction helped alleviate Mr. Thompson's anxiety and instill hope. In health care, patients facing complex information and uncertain outcomes require more than just medical advice; they need someone who truly cares, listens, understands, and supports them throughout their journey. Remember, "Patients don't care how much you know until they know how much you care."

To appreciate the importance of communication, consider the inspiring tale of Sister Elizabeth Kenny and her battle against polio. Back in the early twentieth century, polio was a dreadful illness that terrified parents globally. The conventional treatment recommended by the medical community included immobilizing the patient's impacted limbs with plaster casts or placing them in metal braces. The prevailing notion was immobilization would deter muscle atrophy and deformity. Unfortunately, this approach frequently resulted in significant muscle loss and restricted improvement in muscle functionality.

Elizabeth Kenny was an Australian nurse who perfected her muscle rehabilitation skills during World War I. In civilian life, Kenny treated her first polio patient as a young child in rural Australia. Witnessing the child's intense muscle pain and stiffness, Kenny tried an unconventional approach of hot, moist clothes, which surprisingly relieved the pain. Encouraged by this progress, Kenny delved into various physical therapy methods, incorporating gentle exercises posting hot compresses to aid muscle recovery.

Despite seeing significant progress in her patients, Kenny faced doubt and push-back from the traditional medical field. Some doctors were skeptical and even unfriendly toward a nurse who dared to question established practices. Nevertheless, Kenny remained undeterred by the medical establishment's firm position. She had complete faith in her approach, which focused on observing patient reactions rather than blindly following medical beliefs.

Kenny was determined to promote her treatment approach and took a bold step by traveling to England and then to the United States during polio outbreaks. Despite initial opposition in the United States, she eventually found a platform to demonstrate her techniques. Her persistence resulted in a successful pilot program in Minnesota, where her methods showed clear benefits over traditional treatments, leading to broader adoption. Kenny then focused on training other nurses and therapists in her methods, establishing training centers, and traveling extensively to teach her techniques to others. She emphasized the importance of understanding the patient's experience and actively engaging them in treatment.

Kenny's ability to effectively communicate was crucial. She wrote a lot, delivered lectures, and interacted directly with the medical community and the public to promote her treatment methods. By clearly, compassionately, and assertively explaining the advantages of her approach, she successfully overcame the significant challenges she encountered [11, 16].

Effective communication is crucial for providing patient-centered care. It is a vital link between health care providers and patients, fostering understanding, trust, and successful treatment. Communication in health care goes beyond sharing information; it is about establishing a relationship that helps patients feel valued, heard, and dignified. This chapter explores key elements of effective communication, providing valuable tips and strategies for health care providers to improve patient interactions.

**Table 5.1** Steps to effective communication in medical setups

| | |
|---|---|
| Step 1 | The art of listening |
| Step 2 | Mastering the art of asking questions |
| Step 3 | Understanding nonverbal clues |
| Step 4 | Sharing opinions and information |
| Step 5 | Encouraging and answering patient questions |

## Steps to Effective Communication in Medical Setups

Effective communication in medical setups has five steps (Table 5.1).

## Step 1: The Art of Listening

In health care, listening extends far beyond hearing words; it involves interpreting, understanding, and responding to patients in ways that foster trust and healing. Dr. Rachel Naomi, a renowned doctor, author, and teacher, frequently emphasizes the importance of listening in connecting with others: "The most basic and powerful way to connect to another person is to listen. Just listen. Perhaps the most important thing we ever give each other is our attention" [14]. This attention can mean the difference between life and death, and health and illness in health care.

### Active Listening

Active listening involves more than just hearing words: It requires the listener to fully concentrate, understand, respond, and remember what the speaker is saying. Active listening ensures the speaker feels heard, understood, and valued by being fully engaged verbally and nonverbally.

In health care, active listening aims to connect fully with patients through verbal and nonverbal cues. This method fosters trust, enhances understanding of patient concerns, and improves treatment outcomes.

As an internal medical resident, I worked in the oncology unit, where emotions often ran high, and quiet resignation was not uncommon. One patient in particular left an indelible mark on me. She was a 68-year-old woman diagnosed with advanced pancreatic cancer.

From the moment I met her, she seemed emotionally withdrawn. During morning rounds, she would respond with little more than a nod or a soft "okay." No questions, no complaints—just a quiet acceptance that seemed to mask something more profound. Despite my repeated efforts to offer information and guidance, she remained distant, her eyes dull and tired. Something about her silence lingered in my mind.

One afternoon, as my shift wound down, I lingered outside her room. I had read about the importance of active listening in medical training, but this moment demanded more than clinical skills—it required connection. I decided to step inside.

I pulled a chair beside her bed and asked, "Would it be alright if I sat with you for a bit?"

She looked surprised as if no one had asked her that in a long time. With a faint shrug, she whispered, "Sure."

I took a deep breath and asked a simple, open-ended question: "Can you tell me how you're feeling about everything today?"

For a moment, there was only silence. I wondered if I'd overstepped. But then, her eyes glistened, and her voice, soft yet strained, broke the quiet.

"I'm… scared," she said, her fingers clutching the blanket. "I don't know what's coming next. They keep saying things about chemo and radiation, but… I don't know if I can handle it."

I nodded gently, giving her space. "That sounds overwhelming," I said quietly. "Tell me more about what's been on your mind."

The dam broke. Her words tumbled out—her fears of unrelenting pain, her dread of spending her remaining days too sick to move, her anxiety that her husband wouldn't know how to manage without her. She worried the side effects of chemotherapy would steal whatever time she had left, leaving her bedridden, robbed of dignity, and unable to see her family.

"I just want to have some good days," she said, her voice breaking. "I want to see my grandchildren without being hooked up to machines… I want to sit in my garden again. I don't want my last memories with them to be… like this."

I felt the weight of her words. Instead of rushing in with medical advice, I paused. I could feel how important it was to honor her fears, not fix them.

"I hear you," I said softly. "And I want to help you have those good days. Can we talk about what that might look like?"

Her eyes widened. For the first time, she looked hopeful, like someone had finally seen her, not just her diagnosis. We discussed her priorities—her love for her garden, her longing to spend unburdened time with her family, and her desire to avoid aggressive treatment that would leave her bedridden. Together, we explored ways to adjust her pain management strategy so she could have more moments of comfort and clarity.

By the end of our conversation, her face had softened. "Thank you," she said quietly. "I feel… lighter. Like someone finally understands what I'm terrified of."

That encounter changed my perspective on patient care. I realized patients often carry unspoken burdens—fears they may never articulate unless we create the space for them to do so. Active listening isn't just about hearing words; it's about reading between the lines, giving patients the dignity of sharing their struggles and showing their voice matters.

In this case, active listening didn't just improve our rapport; it reshaped her care. By understanding her priorities, we adjusted her treatment plan to focus on maximizing comfort and creating meaningful time with her loved ones.

This experience taught me a profound lesson: Active listening is as powerful as any prescription in medicine. By pausing, listening, and responding with empathy, we don't just treat illness; we affirm the humanity of those we care for.

Dr. Danielle Ofri, a physician at Bellevue Hospital in New York, has spent much of her career exploring the complexities of doctor-patient communication. In her book *What Patients Say, What Doctors Hear*, she recounts a powerful encounter with Julia, whose story illustrates the profound impact of active listening in clinical care.

Julia was a middle-aged woman battling poorly controlled diabetes. Her medical record painted a troubling picture: repeated missed appointments, unstable blood glucose levels, and a pattern of non-compliance with treatment recommendations. Over time, Julia had earned the frustrating label of being a "difficult patient." Many on the medical team had given up on her, believing she was either unwilling or unable to manage her health.

On one tough afternoon, Julia arrived at the clinic after weeks of missed visits. Her latest test results showed dangerously high glucose levels. As Dr. Ofri read the results, she felt frustration rising—a feeling she knew many of her colleagues had also experienced with Julia. The instinctive reaction was to lecture Julia on the risks of uncontrolled diabetes.

But something made Dr. Ofri pause. She remembered a key lesson from her training: patients often carry invisible burdens. Rather than launching into warnings and medical advice, she set her clipboard down, pulled a chair close, and asked Julia quietly, "Can you tell me what's been going on?"

Julia's expression hardened. Her arms crossed, and she barely met Dr. Ofri's eyes. "I know what you're going to say," she muttered. "I haven't been taking care of myself."

Instead of pushing, Dr. Ofri remained silent, maintaining eye contact. She nodded gently, signaling her willingness to listen, not judge. After a moment, Julia let out a heavy sigh. Her defensive posture softened, and her words flowed.

"My son got arrested," Julia began, her voice trembling. "My husband's out of work, and we're barely keeping things together. I've been picking up extra shifts working doubles just to pay the rent. When I get home, I'm too tired to cook, check my blood glucose, or even think about myself."

Julia's voice broke. "I'm not ignoring my diabetes… I just don't have the energy to deal with it."

Hearing this, Dr. Ofri felt a profound shift. Julia's medical history—her so-called "non-compliance"—wasn't about negligence or carelessness. It was the story of a woman drowning in stress and hardship.

Instead of scolding or advising, Dr. Ofri leaned forward and said softly, "That sounds incredibly hard. I can understand why this feels overwhelming."

Julia's eyes widened in surprise. The frustration that had colored their previous encounters seemed to melt away. For the first time, Julia opened up about her concerns—her fears about her family, her sense of helplessness, and her growing anxiety about her health.

For the next 20 min, Dr. Ofri simply listened. No instructions, no corrections—just quiet, compassionate attention. When Julia finally paused, Dr. Ofri asked, "Would it help if we worked on a manageable plan for you?"

Together, they designed a treatment strategy that reflected Julia's reality. Instead of overwhelming changes, they focused on small, achievable steps: quick, diabetes-friendly meals Julia could prepare even after a long shift, timing her medications to fit her chaotic schedule, and setting realistic goals for exercise. Julia left the clinic that day not just with a plan, but with a sense of control.

Over the following months, Julia returned consistently for her appointments. Her blood glucose levels gradually improved, and her engagement in her care strengthened. Most importantly, she no longer felt judged or dismissed; she felt understood. Reflecting on this encounter, Dr. Ofri wrote: "Listening may be the most powerful diagnostic tool we have" [10].

Julia's story reveals a fundamental truth: Listening is not passive but an active and intentional skill. Active listening can be as powerful as the most sophisticated medical intervention in medicine. By listening with empathy, doctors uncover what's wrong physically and what's preventing patients from achieving better health.

In a world where busy clinics and tight schedules often make deep conversations difficult, Julia's story reminds us that sometimes, the most significant impact comes not from prescribing more medication but simply pulling up a chair and asking, "Can you tell me what's been going on?"

Active listening involves several key behaviors that signal to the patient the health care provider is fully engaged and genuinely interested in their well-being.

1. **Maintain Eye Contact:** Maintaining eye contact is a powerful way to communicate nonverbally. It lets the patient know the health care provider is attentive and genuinely listening. Yet, it's crucial to consider cultural differences and individual comfort levels, as excessive eye contact may be intimidating.
2. **Nod Appropriately:** Nodding is a simple yet effective way to show medical providers are following along with what the patient is saying without interrupting them. It encourages the speaker to continue and conveys that their messages are being received and understood.
3. **Use Verbal Affirmations:** Phrases like "I see," "Go on," or "Tell me more" are verbal nods that can significantly enhance the effectiveness of communication. They reassure the patient that the listener is engaged and interested in hearing more about their thoughts and feelings.
4. **Mirroring:** Reflecting the emotions or words of the patient can show empathy and understanding. Mirroring involves repeating what the patient has said or summarizing their main points, which helps confirm understanding and make the patient feel valued.
5. **Avoid Interruptions:** Allowing the patient to speak without interrupting is crucial in active listening. Interruptions can signal impatience and can lead to a breakdown in communication. Patients often need time to articulate their thoughts and feelings, especially about complex or emotional health issues.

6. **Body Language:** Open and inviting body language (such as leaning slightly forward and keeping arms uncrossed) reinforces engagement. It makes the patient feel more at ease and willing to share important details about their health.

Incorporating active listening into patient interactions takes a bit of practice and awareness. Health care providers should intentionally engage in these behaviors during their consultations. Gathering patient feedback can enhance and tailor active listening techniques to better suit the unique needs of each individual.

During the early twentieth century, industrial laborers in the United States encountered hazardous working conditions that neglected their well-being. They often faced exposure to harmful substances, leading to severe, sometimes deadly, diseases. Dr. Alice Hamilton, the inaugural professor at Harvard Medical School, committed her professional life to transforming this situation.

Dr. Hamilton started her adventure at Hull House in Chicago, a community center where she resided with immigrants and families with low income. By actively listening to the workers share their situations and symptoms, she collected vital information on the health effects of industrial labor. She observed trends of sickness associated with particular sectors, such as lead, mercury, and radium poisoning, among factory workers.

Her approach included communicating with the employees in their native languages to grasp their experiences and symptoms. She was heavily involved in active listening during these interactions. She also carefully recorded details about the industrial procedures and materials. This interactive research method was unusual during that period, particularly for a female professional in her industry. Dr. Hamilton's findings were compelling and led her to advocate for industrial hygiene. She worked tirelessly to raise awareness among policymakers and the public about the dangers of chemical exposure in the workplace. Her ability to actively listen to the complexities of industrial medicine in straightforward, impactful ways was crucial to her success. Her work resulted in some of the first occupational health laws in the United States, transforming how industries addressed worker safety and health [7, 17].

## Reflective Listening

Reflective listening involves actively trying to understand what the speaker is saying by carefully listening and then repeating, summarizing, or reflecting on their words to confirm understanding. This technique prioritizes empathy, clarity, and validation, which helps build trust and improve communication. In health care, reflective listening is a beneficial approach that strengthens the relationship between health care providers and patients.

During my nephrology fellowship, I encountered a case that deeply reinforced the power of reflective listening in fostering patient trust and improving care outcomes. The patient was a 63-year-old man with chronic kidney disease facing the inevitable transition to dialysis. While this was a clinical decision based on clear medical evidence, his strong resistance and anxiety about starting dialysis made the situation increasingly challenging.

For several years, he had managed his condition well through medication, dietary adjustments, and lifestyle changes. However, recent tests revealed his kidney function had deteriorated to a point where dialysis was no longer optional—it was essential for his survival. Despite understanding this medically, he remained adamant that dialysis was not the right choice for him. His concerns went beyond the physical implications; they were deeply emotional and psychological.

One afternoon, I decided to have an open conversation with him. I focused on understanding his perspective instead of leading with medical explanations or facts. I knew that to connect with him, I needed to listen and not just hear his words, but truly understand his feelings. I began with a calm and open question: "Can you tell me what's been worrying you the most about dialysis?"

At first, his response was brief and guarded. He mentioned concerns about "being tied to a machine" and "losing control" over his life. But rather than jumping in with reassurance or counterarguments, I remained silent, allowing him to elaborate. As the silence stretched, he slowly revealed more.

He spoke about his fear of becoming dependent on others—worried that dialysis would strip away his independence. He described deep-seated anxiety about no longer being able to travel, spend time outdoors, or maintain his morning routine of walking his dog—moments that defined his sense of purpose. He also admitted to feeling ashamed, believing dialysis carried a stigma that made him feel weaker or less capable.

I knew this was a pivotal moment. Rather than rushing in with solutions, I paused and reflected on his words to him: "It sounds like you're worried that dialysis will take away your independence and the life you've worked hard to maintain. It seems like you feel dialysis may limit your freedom and leave you feeling helpless. Is that what you're feeling?"

His expression softened. He sighed deeply with a release of tension I hadn't seen before. "Yes," he said quietly. "That's exactly it. I'm scared of losing control over my own life."

That moment shifted everything. By reflecting on his emotions, I had shown him I wasn't just there to dictate a treatment plan; I was there to understand his fears. Encouraged by this validation, he began sharing more openly. He talked about his worries about becoming a burden to his family and his fear of losing his role as the person who always cared for others.

I continued to use reflective listening throughout our conversation, carefully summarizing his concerns and confirming I had understood him correctly. Whenever I reflected on his feelings, he seemed more willing to engage. This approach not only validated his concerns but also created an opportunity for me to address his fears in a meaningful way. For example, after he voiced his concerns about dialysis limiting his ability to travel, I introduced information about peritoneal dialysis, a home-based option that could give him greater flexibility. When he mentioned his worry about social stigma, I offered to connect him with a support group where other patients had shared similar experiences.

By the end of our conversation, his demeanor had changed. While his concerns hadn't vanished, he seemed more open to exploring his options. He agreed to meet with a dialysis nurse for the first time to learn about treatment options tailored to his lifestyle. He even accepted my suggestion to visit a local dialysis center and speak with other patients who had successfully integrated dialysis into their daily lives.

Reflective listening didn't just help him feel heard; it built a critical foundation of trust. That trust allowed us to move from resistance to collaboration, giving him the confidence to make informed decisions about his care. Reflective listening validated his emotions and allowed me to provide meaningful solutions that resonated with his values and priorities.

This experience reinforced an essential truth in medicine: Patients need to feel heard before they can accept guidance. Reflective listening is not just about repeating words; it's about understanding the emotions behind those words. By allowing him to feel seen, respected, and validated, I guided him toward a treatment path that aligned with his values and maintained his sense of independence. In nephrology, a field where patients face lifelong treatment decisions, reflective listening is a powerful tool. It transforms difficult conversations into meaningful partnerships, ensuring care decisions are guided by clinical evidence and the patient's voice.

Reflective listening involves several key steps that health care providers can utilize during patient interactions:

1. **Paraphrasing** entails paraphrasing the patient's statements using the health care provider's terminology. This demonstrates that the provider is attentively listening and comprehending the information provided by the patient. For instance, if a patient mentions, "I become extremely anxious and can't focus before my treatments," the provider could reply, "It appears you experience intense anxiety before your procedures."
2. **Summarizing**: Condensing what the patient has said into a brief overview helps reinforce the discussion and ensure mutual understanding. For example, the provider might say, "In summary, your main concerns are the medication's side effects and its impact on your daily routine, right?"
3. **Asking for Confirmation**: After paraphrasing or summarizing, it is essential to ask the patient if you have understood them correctly. Questions such as "Did I understand that correctly?" or "Is there anything else you would like to mention?" encourage the patient to address any misconceptions and provide additional information if needed.
4. **Emotional Reflecting**: Recognizing the emotions behind the patient's words and mirroring them is an essential aspect of patient care. For example, if a patient feels frustrated and anxious about their diagnosis, the provider can respond by acknowledging, "It sounds like you're finding this uncertainty quite overwhelming."
5. **Silence**: Effective reflective listening also includes allowing pauses and silence after reflecting. This allows the patient to agree, correct, or elaborate further, leading to deeper insights and more effective communication.

## Empathetic Listening

Empathetic listening is a communication technique in which the listener actively engages with the speaker by demonstrating genuine understanding, compassion, and emotional connection. Unlike essential listening, empathetic listening requires the listener to focus not only on the speaker's words but also on their emotions, perspectives, and unspoken concerns.

Empathetic listening goes beyond hearing information; it involves putting oneself in the speaker's shoes and responding with sensitivity and care. The goal is to create a safe environment where the speaker feels acknowledged, valued, and understood.

Abraham Lincoln is widely respected as one of the most remarkable leaders in American history. He had a unique talent for connecting with people by listening empathetically. This skill was crucial to his leadership, particularly during the challenging times of the American Civil War. Lincoln ensured wounded soldiers were personally visited in hospitals during the war. These visits were more than just quick formalities; Lincoln would spend considerable time talking with soldiers, sometimes sitting quietly by their bedside to hear their fears, sorrows, and personal tales. His presence brought solace during a period of doubt and hopelessness.

One touching instance of Lincoln's empathetic listening occurred during a military hospital visit. A Union soldier, not realizing he was speaking to the President, shared his sadness about not being able to see his family again and worried about the impact of his death on his loved ones. Instead of offering patriotic speeches, Lincoln sat by his side, held his hand, and asked about his life. By asking the soldier about his home, family, and comforting memories, he helped the soldier shift from despair to reminiscing about the warmth of home. Lincoln's quiet and empathetic presence comforted the soldier in his final moments, showing a rare and deeply human side of a leader carrying the nation's weight.

This decisive moment reflects a core principle of Lincoln's leadership—the belief that understanding others' emotions was crucial to guiding people through hardship. Lincoln knew genuine connection required listening without judgment and responding with empathy. Historians have highlighted Lincoln's emotional intelligence as a defining feature of his leadership. As Doris Kearns Goodwin notes in *Team of Rivals,* Lincoln's ability to "acknowledge the burdens of others with patience and empathy allowed him to forge powerful alliances and maintain public trust during the nation's darkest hours" [6].

Lincoln's demonstration of empathetic listening highlighted the essence of successful leadership, which goes beyond making decisions. It emphasizes acknowledging the emotional burden carried by others. His ability to console the dying soldier with understanding and empathy, rather than elaborate speeches, remains a timeless example of empathetic listening during moments of vulnerability [2, 13].

Developing empathetic listening skills requires attention, intention, and practice. The following techniques can enhance the ability to connect with others empathetically:

1. **Active Presence**: Being completely focused is crucial for good empathetic listening. This involves reducing distractions, making eye contact, and concentrating entirely on the patients. Following these steps shows that you are fully engaged in the discussion. Nonverbal signals like nodding, leaning in, and keeping an open body posture also show attentiveness. These subtle gestures indicate you are listening attentively and value what the speaker is saying.
2. **Identify Emotional Cues**: It's essential to pay attention to emotional cues to better understand how the patient is feeling. These cues can be found in the patient's tone of voice, pace of speech, and choice of words. For example, speaking quickly with a raised tone might indicate feelings of anxiety or being overwhelmed. Conversely, a quiet voice with frequent pauses could signal sadness or uncertainty. Recognizing these signals helps you grasp the emotions underlying their words.
3. **Acknowledge Emotions**: Acknowledging the patient's emotions is a powerful method to validate their experience. Using phrases such as, "It seems like you're feeling…" or "I understand this situation has been tough for you," provide comfort and show empathy. Moreover, prompting more discussion with statements like, "I feel that you're frustrated. Do you want to discuss it further?" fosters deeper conversation and assures the speaker their feelings are recognized.
4. **Resist the Urge to Fix**: Empathetic listening involves not rushing to offer solutions unless asked. Instead of giving advice immediately, concentrate on grasping the patient's emotions. It's important to remember that sometimes, individuals just need to share their thoughts and feel understood. Refraining from trying to solve their issues immediately creates a supportive environment for them to fully explore their feelings and ideas.
5. **Silence as a Tool**: Silence can be powerful in empathetic listening. Avoid the urge to fill pauses or interrupt the patient. Allowing moments of silence gives the patient time to reflect, process their emotions, and continue the conversation at their own pace. These quiet moments encourage the patient to open up further, deepening the connection and fostering greater understanding.

## Step 2: Mastering the Art of Asking Questions

Mastering the skill of effective questioning is crucial for patient-centered communication. Asking thoughtful and strategic questions can reveal important information, enhance diagnostic accuracy, and nurture better medical provider-patient connections. Achieving proficiency in this area involves recognizing different question types and being emotionally sensitive.

Sir William Osler (1849–1919) is often hailed as the father of modern medicine for his patient-centered approach that transformed medical education and clinical practice. He believed effective questioning was crucial for accurate diagnosis and building strong doctor-patient relationships. Osler's adept use of detailed patient dialogue distinguished him as a diagnostician and influenced modern clinical examination practices. One notable instance showcasing Osler's diagnostic prowess was when he successfully diagnosed a patient with chronic poisoning due to occupational exposure by delving into their lifestyle and work environment through thoughtful questioning.

This example highlights Osler's firm belief that a patient's story is crucial for making a diagnosis. His famous quote, "Listen to your patient; he is telling you the diagnosis," sums up this idea. By actively listening and asking the right questions, Osler consistently showed that effective communication could provide insights that tests and imaging might overlook. Osler's focus on questioning wasn't limited to individual cases but was a central part of his teaching style. He encouraged medical students to spend time with patients, attentively listening to their stories and understanding their worries. He famously said, "The good physician treats the disease; the great physician treats the patient who has the disease." This method emphasized the significance of grasping the patient's social, emotional, and environmental background—aspects that often surface through thoughtful questioning.

Modern scholars emphasize Osler's impact on medical communication. Dr. Michael Bliss, Osler's biographer, notes Osler's clinical expertise was closely linked to his talent for eliciting information from patients through empathetic questioning, a skill that shaped his legacy [1]. Dr. Abraham Verghese also underscores Osler's teachings in current medical practice, highlighting that unraveling the patient's narrative through adept questioning remains a crucial diagnostic tool in the modern era [19].

Osler's method is still highly pertinent today. His skill in asking the right questions is a timeless lesson emphasizing the importance of the patient's story and medical knowledge. Through attentive listening and thoughtful questioning, health care professionals can reveal essential details, build trust, and enhance patient results—a principle that continues to influence contemporary medical care.

## Types of Questions in Medical Practice

It is important for medical professionals to grasp various question types and how to use them strategically. The subsequent categories demonstrate the effective application of these questions.

1. **Open-Ended Questions**

   Open-ended questions are a great tool in clinical communication. They encourage patients to share their perspectives and provide detailed responses, unlike closed-ended questions that elicit short answers. Patients can describe their symptoms, concerns, and experiences in their own words, helping medical providers gather comprehensive information for diagnosis and treatment. Asking patients to describe their pain or concerns can reveal insights that might otherwise be overlooked, especially in cases with complex symptoms. Open-ended questions are valuable at the start of a consultation to build a connection and allow patients to express their main concerns. They can also address hidden issues affecting the patient's condition. Using prompts like "What...," "How...," or "Tell me about…" can make open-ended questions more effective by promoting conversation and showing patients they are being listened to and respected. Health care providers can discover important information that enhances diagnosis and strengthens the doctor-patient bond by listening to the patient's story.

2. **Closed-Ended Questions**

   Closed-ended questions are also essential in medical communication as they help gather specific information quickly. They are valuable for verifying details, collecting accurate data, and clarifying information. By prompting clear and concise answers, closed-ended questions assist clinicians in efficiently obtaining necessary facts for diagnosis and treatment. However, balancing their use with open-ended questions is important to encourage deeper dialogue. This approach helps establish trust, ensures thorough information gathering, and supports patient-centered care.

3. **Probing Questions**

   Probing questions are a vital communication tool in health care that encourages patients to think more deeply about their answers or provide additional details. These questions help uncover specific information that can enhance our understanding of a patient's experiences or symptoms. For instance, asking, "You mentioned feeling anxious—can you share more about that?" fosters a conversation that allows patients to express their feelings and concerns in greater depth. Likewise, asking, "What do you mean when you say the pain 'comes and goes'?" invites patients to explain the pattern or intensity of their symptoms, which is essential for accurate diagnosis and treatment planning. Probing questions are beneficial when a patient's response is unclear or needs further clarification to ensure we provide the best care.

4. **Reflective Questions**

   Reflective questions are a great way to help patients delve into their thoughts, feelings, and insights regarding their health. These questions promote self-reflection and encourage active involvement in decision-making. For example, asking, "How do you feel about your treatment plan?" allows patients to consider their comfort levels and any concerns they might have. Likewise, questions like "What do you think will help you manage your condition better?" empower patients to discover strategies that resonate with them, giving them a sense of ownership over their health journey. Reflective questions are especially beneficial when discussing lifestyle changes, coping strategies, or long-term health goals, as they steer patients toward finding personal motivation and solutions for managing their condition.

5. **Hypothetical Questions**

   Hypothetical questions are a fantastic way to enhance communication in health care. They allow patients to think about possible outcomes and explore various solutions or scenarios. These questions are great for understanding a patient's preferences, concerns, and readiness for future decisions. For instance, asking, "If your symptoms worsen, what would you like to do next?" helps patients consider their options and mentally prepare for any changes in their condition. Likewise, "If surgery becomes necessary, how do you feel about that option?" encourages patients to think about their comfort level with more invasive treatments. These questions are beneficial when discussing treatment plans, potential complications, or future steps, as they help gauge patient understanding, reduce anxiety, and promote proactive decision-making.

6. **Clarifying Questions**

   Clarification questions are crucial in medical communication, especially when patients express symptoms unclearly. By asking questions like, "When you mention 'dizzy,' are you referring to feeling lightheaded or a spinning sensation?" or "Could you explain what you mean by 'feeling off'?" health care professionals can ensure they fully grasp the patient's situation. These questions are vital in resolving confusion caused by medical terms or vague language, helping to bridge communication gaps and steer clinicians toward accurate diagnoses and effective treatment plans. Seeking clarification shows empathy, enhances relationships, and reduces the chance of misunderstandings in clinical care.

7. **Empathic Questions**

   Empathetic questions are a valuable resource in medical conversations. They help to show care, acknowledge feelings, and establish trust with patients. Questions like, "How has this been affecting your daily life?" or "I imagine this must be difficult for you—how are you coping?" demonstrate empathy and encourage patients to share their worries. These questions are especially beneficial when talking about delicate topics such as long-term illnesses, mental health issues, or social difficulties. By recognizing the patient's emotions, health care providers develop a stronger bond, improving comprehension and teamwork in the treatment journey.

A remarkable historical example that highlights the importance of using different types of questions in clinical practice is the story of Dr. Barry Marshall and the discovery of *Helicobacter pylori* as the cause of peptic ulcers.

During the 1980s, the medical community commonly believed stress, spicy foods, and too much stomach acid were the main culprits behind peptic ulcers. Patients with persistent ulcers were typically advised to take antacids, follow dietary restrictions, and manage stress. However, despite these treatments, many patients still experienced discomfort. During this challenging situation, Dr. Barry Marshall, an Australian doctor and pathologist, and Dr. Robin Warren challenged these established beliefs.

Marshall's journey began with curiosity sparked by Warren's discovery of spiral-shaped bacteria in stomach biopsies from patients with gastritis. Rather than accepting the prevailing explanations, Marshall asked a pivotal open-ended question: "*What if the bacteria are causing the ulcers?*"

This question challenged decades of established medical thought. Marshall's willingness to explore an unconventional idea opened new pathways in ulcer research.

As he delved deeper, Marshall employed probing questions to investigate patient histories more thoroughly. He asked patients detailed questions like:

"When do your symptoms worsen?" "Have you noticed any changes in your symptoms after taking antibiotics?"

By combining these probing questions with careful observation, Marshall identified a pattern: many ulcer patients had signs of bacterial infection, particularly from a previously overlooked microbe, later identified as Helicobacter pylori. This discovery was revolutionary because it contradicted the belief that ulcers were stress-induced.

Marshall further employed clarifying questions to distinguish between different gastrointestinal symptoms. He asked patients to describe their pain—burning, cramping, or sharp? Did it worsen on an empty stomach or after eating? These distinctions helped him connect specific ulcer patterns with the presence of H. pylori, advancing his hypothesis.

During his research, Marshall also recognized the emotional toll that long-term ulcers impose on patients. Many felt helpless after years of ineffective treatments. By asking empathic questions like: "*How has this condition been affecting your daily life?*" he created space for patients to share their frustrations. This strengthened trust and encouraged patients to collaborate actively in their care.

Perhaps the most dramatic moment in this medical journey came when Marshall posed a hypothetical question to himself: "*If no one believes this bacterium causes ulcers, what would happen if I infected myself with it?*"

In 1984, in a bold and unconventional move, Marshall drank a culture of H. pylori to prove his theory. Within days, he developed severe gastritis, symptoms mirroring those experienced by his patients. He successfully treated himself through antibiotics, further validating the link between H. pylori *and* peptic ulcers.

Marshall's strategic use of open-ended, probing, clarifying, empathic, and hypothetical questioning ultimately transformed the medical understanding of ulcers. In 2005, he and Warren were awarded the Nobel Prize in Physiology for their groundbreaking discovery.

Marshall's journey highlights the importance of asking the right questions in medicine. By questioning assumptions, delving into patient experiences, and considering hypothetical situations, he transformed ulcer treatment and saved many lives. His experience shows that timely, insightful questions can lead to significant discoveries, advance science, and enhance patient care [9].

As an internal medicine resident, I witnessed a moment that solidified the importance of asking the right questions in clinical practice. One afternoon, we were rounding with one of my attendings, and we encountered a patient with a long-standing history of vague symptoms—fatigue, joint pain, and digestive issues. The patient had visited multiple specialists over the years, but no one could pinpoint the cause.

As we gathered around the bedside, my attending began asking questions that immediately struck me. Instead of diving into closed-ended questions that might only elicit brief responses, he started with an open-ended one: "Can you describe a typical day for you? When do you feel the most discomfort?"

I watched as the patient paused momentarily, visibly surprised by the question. She began sharing not just her symptoms but the emotional and mental toll it had taken on her life. It was clear the patient had been struggling in silence, never fully able to articulate the depth of her experience. The open-ended question had given her the space to express her feelings, something no other doctor had done before.

But my attending didn't stop there. He followed up with a probing question, "You mentioned your pain is worse in the mornings—can you describe how it feels?" The patient responded with more detail than before, explaining how the pain in her joints wasn't just stiffness but a burning sensation that worsened after waking up. I could see how this question helped him uncover a pattern that could point toward an autoimmune condition.

Then, the attending asked a clarifying question, which was something I hadn't considered: "When you say you're 'feeling off,' can you elaborate on what that means?" The patient explained it wasn't just physical discomfort but a sense of disconnection from her body, a heaviness that clouded their ability to function normally. Clarifying her response was crucial for a more accurate understanding of the case.

Noticing the emotional burden this patient carried, my attending asked an empathic question: "How has this been affecting your daily life?" I could see the patient's eyes well up as she shared her frustrations—how it affected her ability to care for her family, work, and even enjoy simple activities. This wasn't just a case of physical illness; it was affecting her whole life, and my attending acknowledged that with sensitivity.

Finally, the attending posed a hypothetical question: "If we find out this is something like lupus, would you be open to starting a treatment plan for that?" This question allowed the patient to process what might come next, to mentally prepare for potential treatments, and to express any concerns or reservations. It helped gauge her readiness for the next steps in care.

As I watched this unfold, it became clear how effectively my attending used different types of questions to gather a comprehensive understanding of the patient's condition. Not only did he uncover critical diagnostic information, but he also showed deep empathy and respect for the patient's experience. The entire approach fostered a stronger doctor-patient relationship, and it was a powerful lesson for me on the importance of asking the right questions in the right way.

That day, I learned clinical excellence isn't just about knowing; it's about communicating with patients and using questions to guide the conversation. Whether it's an open-ended question to let them share their story, a probing question to dig deeper, or an empathic question to show you care, the right questions can open doors to better diagnoses and care. I carried this lesson with me throughout my residency and continue to use it in practice.

Mastering the skill of asking questions is vital for every medical provider. By skillfully blending open-ended, empathic, and probing inquiries, providers can obtain more valuable information, build stronger relationships, and enhance patient outcomes. Asking the right questions with curiosity, compassion, and respect is not merely a skill but a meaningful expression of care.

## Step 3: Understanding Nonverbal Clues

In the realm of health care, excellent communication involves more than just words. Nonverbal signals—like body language, facial expressions, tone of voice, and eye contact—are essential to the relationship between medical providers and patients. These subtle hints can offer important insights into a patient's condition, feelings, and comfort level with the treatment journey.

1. **Body Language**: A patient's posture can reveal much about their emotional state. For instance, crossed arms might show they feel defensive, uncomfortable, or resistant, while slouched shoulders could indicate fatigue or sadness. On the other hand, open body language often reflects a readiness to connect and trust the doctor. By paying attention to these signals, health care providers can tailor their approach to help patients feel more comfortable or identify when someone might be concealing their true feelings or worries.
2. **Facial Expressions**: The face is commonly seen as a "window to the soul." A patient's facial expressions can convey feelings that words sometimes cannot. For example, a furrowed brow might indicate confusion, worry, or discomfort. Similarly, a smile can be a source of comfort, but it might also hide feelings of anxiety or fear. By being sensitive to these facial cues, medical providers can better understand the emotions patients may find difficult to express verbally.
3. **Tone of Voice**: How we say things can be just as meaningful as the words themselves. A flat or monotone voice might signal depression, tiredness, or low energy, while a lively or faster pace could indicate anxiety or excitement. The tone of voice often adds extra context to what a patient says, especially if they feel shy or uneasy about sharing their deeper feelings.
4. **Eye Contact**: Eye contact is crucial in building trust and connection. In a clinical environment, it can reveal a patient's level of engagement, anxiety, or even if they're holding back. When someone avoids eye contact, it might suggest they're uncomfortable or scared, whereas maintaining eye contact for too long could indicate anxiety or a desire to assert control. For medical providers, recognizing these cues can be invaluable in tailoring their approach—offering reassurance, calming the patient's nerves, or giving them more space.
5. **Physical Symptoms**: Nonverbal cues include physical signs like sweating, pacing, or fidgeting. These behaviors can signal pain, nervousness, or emotions, such as stress or discomfort. By noticing these physical expressions, a medical provider can be encouraged to ask additional questions or suggest ways to manage a patient's anxiety or pain better.
6. **Cultural Sensitivity**: It's worth mentioning that nonverbal signals can differ quite a bit from one culture to another. For instance, in some cultures, keeping eye contact is viewed as a sign of attentiveness and respect; in others, it might be seen as impolite. Being aware of these cultural differences can help prevent misunderstandings and ensure our communication is effective and respectful.

Sigmund Freud, a key figure in medicine and psychology, transformed our understanding of human behavior. His innovative work in psychoanalysis brought forth a way to interpret not only the words of patients but also the insights their bodies, gestures, and facial expressions provided. Freud's keen observation and interpretation of nonverbal signals established the groundwork for much of today's knowledge in human psychology and communication.

In the late nineteenth and early twentieth centuries, Freud embarked on a journey to delve into the deeper layers of the human mind, believing they were shaped by unconscious forces. During that era, patients with psychological issues would typically sit face-to-face with their doctors or therapists, discussing their symptoms, thoughts, and memories. However, Freud introduced a distinctive way of observing patients. Instead of focusing solely on his patients' words, he keenly observed their physical cues, behaviors, and reactions. He paid special attention to unconscious gestures, facial expressions, body language, and changes in posture—those subtle, often involuntary movements that could convey far more than words alone.

Freud observed that while patients might discuss their childhood or distressing memories calmly, their body language—such as a furrowed brow, fidgeting, or avoiding eye contact—revealed a much deeper emotional struggle. He believed these physical signs of the unconscious mind were essential for uncovering the hidden motivations behind their spoken words. A slight change in posture, a nervous chuckle, or a sudden sigh could provide insights into unexpressed feelings, fears, or desires. By paying close attention to these cues, Freud developed the "talking cure," a therapeutic method centered on verbal communication greatly enriched by these nonverbal signals.

Freud's well-known "free association" technique beautifully illustrates the importance of nonverbal communication in his practice. He invited patients to express themselves openly and without limits, allowing their thoughts to flow freely. Throughout these sessions, he keenly observed how their spoken words matched or clashed with their body language and facial expressions. For example, a patient might appear calm while sharing a distressing memory, yet they could hint at their true feelings through subtle actions, such as clenching their fists or avoiding eye contact. These nonverbal cues highlighted emotional tensions that went more profound than the spoken words, often uncovering repressed thoughts or feelings crucial to the patient's challenges.

One of the most well-known examples of this concept is the case of "Anna O," a young woman who experienced various symptoms like paralysis, hallucinations, and intense anxiety. Unfortunately, traditional medical treatments didn't help her much. However, during her therapy with Freud's colleague, Josef Breuer, they discovered that when Anna O. talked about certain distressing events from her past, her symptoms would often ease for a while. Breuer also noted her nonverbal signals—like her facial expressions and physical reactions—as she recounted her traumatic experiences. Eventually, they understood her symptoms were tied to deeply buried emotions and memories. This case played a crucial role in shaping Freud's psychoanalysis, where nonverbal communication, including physical symptoms and emotional reactions, was seen as a reflection of unconscious conflicts.

Freud's research showed that nonverbal communication can be crucial in revealing the hidden emotions, thoughts, and fears patients might struggle to express. His innovative clinical methods transformed psychology and psychiatry while influencing the medical field. Freud's understanding of nonverbal cues helped pave the way for more comprehensive patient care, emphasizing that grasping a patient's emotional and psychological well-being is as vital as addressing their physical symptoms [4, 5, 8].

Fast forward to today, and the insights from Freud's work remain significant in medical practice. Nonverbal communication isn't merely an interesting topic—it's a vital tool for diagnosing and treating patients. As health care professionals, being attuned to the nuances of body language, facial expressions, and tone of voice enhances our ability to connect with patients, helping us identify concerns that might not be immediately clear from their words alone. Contemporary research in health care supports Freud's early findings, demonstrating nonverbal cues play a crucial role in building rapport with patients, enhancing clinical outcomes, and nurturing trust in the doctor-patient relationship.

## Step 4: Sharing Opinions and Information

Ensuring effective communication in medical practice is vital. Health care providers must convey complex medical details in a clear and comforting manner to promote patient well-being. Utilizing various communication strategies like medical terms, analogies, and simplified explanations is key to enhancing clarity, trust, and teamwork in patient care.

1. **Using Medical Jargon Effectively**

Medical terminology is crucial for health care professionals to communicate effectively about conditions and treatments. However, using this language with patients can be overwhelming. Clinicians need to strike a balance by explaining things in a way patients can easily understand. Good clinicians adapt their communication style to match each patient's needs.

When you use medical terms, it's helpful to immediately explain them in plain language. For example, if we say, "You have hypertension," we can add, "That means your blood pressure is consistently too high, which strains your heart and other organs." This kind of translation fosters trust and clarity. It's also good to limit unfamiliar terms in one conversation. Analogies, visuals, and asking patients to repeat what they've heard—the "teach-back" method—can be effective tools to ensure clear communication. Ultimately, the aim is not only to inform but to empower.

2. **Using Analogies in Communication**

Analogies can be incredibly effective when medical providers explain complicated medical ideas to patients. They work by connecting unfamiliar concepts to something the patient already knows. Instead of listing technical facts, medical providers can paint a picture. For instance, to explain a blood clot, they might say, "Think of your blood vessels like a highway—if a clot forms, it's like a traffic jam blocking cars from passing through." That simple mental image helps the patient understand the seriousness of a blockage without needing to know the medical jargon.

Visual analogies can be even more powerful. Take insulin, for example—a provider might describe it as a key that unlocks doors on cells to let sugar in. They might also compare the body's maintenance needs to keeping a car running smoothly or a garden needing care. What matters most is choosing familiar and meaningful comparisons for each patient. Tailoring the analogy to what the patient knows makes the explanation clearer and more personal, and that's when proper understanding happens.

3. **Simplifying Complex Information**

Complex medical information can be overwhelming, especially when patients have a new diagnosis or serious health concerns. Simplifying how information is presented can significantly impact their ability to absorb and understand it. Medical providers can help by breaking things down into smaller, focused conversations. Start with the essentials—the diagnosis, what it means, the proposed treatment plan, and immediate next steps. Once that foundation is set, additional details can be introduced gradually, allowing patients to ask questions and process what they've heard.

It's crucial to use simple, everyday language in health care communication. Rather than medical jargon, using words patients can easily understand is more effective. For instance, instead of stating, "The patient presents with an acute exacerbation of COPD," it's clearer to explain, "Your chronic lung condition has worsened recently, making it more difficult for you to breathe." Brief, focused explanations addressing the patient's essential information help prevent confusion. The aim is not to oversimplify the medical details but to ensure patients can comprehend and engage with their care effectively.

## Visual Aids in Patient Education

Visual aids are valuable for health care professionals seeking to enhance patient education. Visual tools, ranging from simple diagrams to digital animations, help simplify complex medical information and make it easier for patients to comprehend. By providing a visual representation of the body's processes, these aids can alleviate anxiety and empower patients to make well-informed decisions, bridging the gap between medical knowledge and patient understanding.

Diagrams and charts are often utilized in health care settings to clarify anatomy and disease processes. For example, a labeled diagram of the kidney can assist a patient in comprehending the location of their issue and the potential benefits of a transplant. Flowcharts and decision trees are particularly beneficial for explaining treatment choices, as they simplify each stage of the process. These resources are especially valuable when patients learn about disease advancement, like cancer stages or chronic illness timelines, and how prompt treatment can impact results.

In addition to traditional visuals, physical models are commonly used to illustrate intricate anatomical structures. During an explanation, holding a 3D model of organs, such as the heart or kidney, can enhance understanding and make the information more tangible. Some models are interactive, allowing patients to explore systems like the GI tract or blood vessels firsthand, which can significantly aid in comprehending treatment processes. These interactive tools enable patients to actively participate in their diagnosis in a more impactful manner. Digital tools have further advanced these capabilities. Animated videos depicting procedures, mobile apps for medication management, and telemedicine platforms that utilize diagrams and virtual whiteboards all contribute to improved communication. Infographics are also effective, especially for summarizing treatment plans or preventive care. A well-crafted infographic can simplify a complex regimen into visually intuitive steps. Whether in-person or online, visual aids enhance message clarity and help patients feel more confident about their health care.

Dr. Edward Jenner is best known for developing the smallpox vaccine, a groundbreaking achievement that laid the foundation for modern immunology. Born in 1749 in Gloucestershire, England, Jenner grew up when smallpox was one of the most deadly diseases. The disease killed millions of people worldwide, and despite many attempts at treatment, there was no effective cure. The medical community was grappling with ways to prevent its spread, but no one had developed a consistent, safe, and effective method of protection.

Jenner's discovery came about after observing an interesting piece of folk knowledge. In rural England, milkmaids seemed immune to smallpox, a phenomenon passed down through generations. The theory was that the milkmaids who contracted cowpox—a less dangerous disease—did not contract smallpox later in life. Jenner hypothesized that exposure to cowpox, a disease closely related to smallpox, could confer immunity to the more deadly illness.

In 1796, Jenner famously tested this hypothesis on an 8-year-old boy named James Phipps. Jenner inoculated Phipps with matter from a cowpox sore and later exposed him to smallpox. Remarkably, Phipps did not develop the disease. This was the first successful demonstration of vaccination, and it was a moment that changed the course of medicine. However, while Jenner's experiment demonstrated the effectiveness of the vaccine, communicating this discovery to the medical community—and to the public—was an entirely different challenge.

At the time of Jenner's discovery, medical understanding of disease transmission and immunity was still in its infancy. The scientific community had no concept of germs or viruses as we know them today. The idea that exposure to a less dangerous form of disease could prevent a more deadly one was not only revolutionary but also counterintuitive to many. Traditional medical treatments of the time were based on humoral theory (the idea that disease was caused by imbalances in the body's fluids), and the concept of vaccination was a foreign one.

Jenner faced the challenge of proving the efficacy of his discovery and persuading a skeptical medical community and the general public to adopt this novel and untested approach. The key to Jenner's success was his ability to communicate his findings effectively through written work and personal persuasion.

In 1798, Jenner published his findings in a pamphlet titled "An Inquiry into the Causes and Effects of the Variolae Vaccinae," in which he explained his observations and the process of vaccination. The pamphlet was meticulously written, detailing his experiments, the scientific rationale behind immunization, and the results of his trials. Jenner's use of clear, logical, and evidence-based arguments helped establish the credibility of his work.

Moreover, Jenner made an effort to use accessible language. Although his audience included the medical community and the general public, Jenner avoided excessive medical jargon that could confuse or alienate non-experts. He focused instead on the practical aspects of his discovery of how it could prevent disease and save lives.

One of Jenner's most effective strategies for communicating the importance of vaccination was his use of personal testimony. He gathered and published accounts from individuals who had undergone the procedure and been protected from smallpox. Using real-life examples of success, Jenner demonstrated the immediate benefits of vaccination, making it more tangible for his audience. His ability to translate a complex scientific concept into a simple, understandable practice was crucial in the widespread acceptance of vaccination.

In addition to scientific communication, Jenner understood the importance of public education. Smallpox was a disease that affected everyone, and for vaccination to be effective on a larger scale, the public had to be persuaded to accept the procedure. Jenner's ability to communicate directly with the general population was as critical as his work with medical professionals.

Jenner sought to demonstrate the safety of vaccination through public inoculations. One of his most notable public demonstrations was in 1800, when he vaccinated several children from a local village and then exposed them to smallpox to prove they were protected. These visible demonstrations of the safety and effectiveness of vaccination went a long way toward allaying fears and misconceptions.

Jenner also used visual aids, such as illustrations in his pamphlets, to depict the difference between cowpox and smallpox lesions. These images helped clarify the process and show patients exactly what they could expect during the vaccination. By pairing detailed scientific explanations with accessible visual cues, Jenner enhanced understanding and increased the likelihood of public acceptance.

Jenner didn't simply rely on his efforts to spread the word about vaccination; he actively worked with other physicians, public health officials, and advocates to promote his discovery. He used networks of colleagues to share his findings and encourage vaccination. Jenner's advocacy also extended to the royal family, and his work gained the support of King George III, who endorsed vaccination publicly, lending it credibility and visibility.

Jenner's ability to communicate through multiple channels—scientific publications, public demonstrations, visual aids, and advocacy—played a key role in the rapid spread of vaccination. His success was not just in discovering the vaccine but also in how effectively he communicated its benefits to a wide range of audiences.

Dr. Edward Jenner's story is a powerful example of how effective communication can influence the course of medical history. His ability to explain a complex new concept in accessible and compelling ways to both medical professionals and the public was instrumental in making vaccination a widely accepted practice. Jenner's clear communication helped save millions of lives and has impacted public health policy and global immunization efforts [15].

Just as Jenner bridged scientific innovation with public understanding, I began to see how vital clear communication is in my own practice—especially when guiding patients through the complexities of kidney transplantation.

While working as a transplant nephrologist, I learned from an attending physician who taught me an invaluable technique for explaining complex transplant concepts to patients. One of the most important aspects of my role is helping patients understand their options with kidney transplants. These options typically include living donor kidneys, deceased donor kidneys, and deceased donor kidneys with a high Kidney Donor Profile Index (KDPI), which essentially refers to kidneys that may be of lower quality due to various factors such as age, underlying health conditions, prolonged cold ischemic time, or prior organ damage.

Initially, I found it challenging to communicate these intricate details to patients who often felt overwhelmed by the medical jargon. That's when my attending shared an approach that made all the difference—using simple analogies to break down complicated concepts. He explained that when discussing these types of kidneys, it could be helpful to compare the situation to something as familiar as buying a car.

I adopted his analogy, and it truly resonated with my patients. A living donor kidney, for example, is like buying a brand-new car. It's fresh, untouched, and in its prime condition. It's the ideal option, as it provides the best long-term outcomes for the patient, just like a brand-new car offers the most reliability. A kidney from a deceased donor, which is of good quality, could be compared to purchasing a car with around 50,000 to 60,000 miles on it. It's not new, but it's still in great shape and can serve you well for many years.

The real challenge comes when we discuss kidneys with a high KDPI, which often leaves patients feeling uncertain about the decision. This is where the analogy becomes even more helpful: I liken it to buying a car with over 100,000 miles. While it may still function, the vehicle (or kidney) is more likely to need repairs or replacement sooner than the other options. It's not necessarily a bad choice, but it comes with the understanding that more risks may be involved.

This simple analogy makes it easier for patients to grasp the different types of donor kidneys and their associated risks. My attending taught me that, while the medical details are important, sometimes it's the most straightforward explanations that allow patients to feel more comfortable and informed when making life-changing decisions. By comparing kidney quality to a situation they are familiar with, like buying a car, patients are empowered to make proper decisions based on their values and preferences. This method has proven to be one of the most effective ways I've learned to communicate with patients and ensure they fully understand the transplant process.

Effective communication goes beyond just sharing medical facts; it's about helping patients genuinely understand that information so they can make informed decisions. Using analogies, simplifying complex ideas, and providing clear visual aids are key skills in this process. These techniques help health care professionals remove the obstacles of medical jargon and complicated concepts, making information more accessible. This boosts patient understanding and strengthens the bond between patients and health care providers, building trust and improving outcomes. Mastering these communication skills is vital for any health care professional to ensure patients feel heard, informed, and engaged in their health care journey.

## Step 5: Encouraging and Answering Patient Questions

As health care professionals, our responsibilities go beyond just diagnosing and treating health issues; we also aim to build understanding and trust with our patients. One of the most effective ways to establish this trust is by encouraging patients to ask questions. This practice is crucial for the quality of care they receive and for enhancing the relationship between patients and doctors.

For many patients, being in a medical environment can be quite daunting. Whether in an emergency department, outpatient clinic, or inpatient unit, the overwhelming amount of information, medical jargon, and the often-critical nature of the situation can leave them feeling vulnerable, confused, and disconnected. We can make a difference by encouraging patients to voice their concerns and ask questions. This approach empowers patients to take charge of their health and creates a space where they feel heard, understood, and respected.

### The Importance of Encouraging Questions, Big or Small

Patients come from various backgrounds and have different levels of health literacy. Some are familiar with medical terminology, while others might find basic concepts challenging. We need to create an environment where every patient feels comfortable asking questions, no matter how small they might think they are. Unfortunately, many health care providers unintentionally discourage inquiries by dismissing concerns or responding in a way that makes patients feel their questions are insignificant. This can lead to misunderstandings, anxiety, and frustration.

Encouraging even the smallest questions fosters better conversations. It invites patients to share doubts or uncertainties regarding their diagnosis, treatment options, or what lies ahead. This is vital in preventing scenarios where a patient leaves an appointment unclear about important aspects of their care. When patients feel at ease asking questions about medication dosages, possible side effects, or procedural details, they gain a sense of control over their health choices. They transition from being passive recipients of care to active participants in their health journey.

## The Behavioral Techniques to Encourage Questions

Several behavioral techniques can be employed to encourage patients to ask questions, which is key to creating a safe and supportive environment:

1. **Open-ended prompts**: Open-ended questions like "What questions do you have about your treatment plan?" or "How are you feeling about our discussion today?" encourage patients to share their thoughts, concerns, or uncertainties. This method allows patients to participate in the conversation more fully without the pressure of having their questions fit into a specific structure or definition.
2. **Creating a welcoming atmosphere**: Both verbal and nonverbal signals make patients feel at ease when they want to ask questions. Keeping eye contact, speaking in a friendly and welcoming tone, and sitting at eye level (instead of standing above the patient) can help create a friendlier atmosphere. This shows patients that health care providers are approachable, ready to listen, and open to their questions.
3. **Validating their questions**: Every patient's question should be treated respectfully. Acknowledge that their questions are valid, no matter how minor they may seem. For example, after a patient asks a question, providers could say, "That's an important question" or "I'm glad you asked that." Validating questions makes the patient feel valued and heard, which, in turn, encourages them to ask more.
4. **Allowing time for questions**: It's perfectly normal for patients to take a moment to gather their thoughts or feel at ease before asking questions. Make sure to take time during the conversation and avoid interrupting them. At the end of the appointment, it's helpful for providers to pause and say, "Is there anything else you'd like to ask?" Allowing patients the time to digest the information and providing them with an opportunity to ask more questions helps ensure they leave without any lingering doubts.
5. **Reassuring the patient that no question is too small**: It's important to reassure patients that every question, no matter how small, is valued and can help ease any doubts they might have. By letting them know their questions are a vital part of their care journey, you encourage them to share openly. Phrases like "Feel free to ask anything, even if it seems minor" can create a welcoming atmosphere for a more engaging conversation.

## The Importance of Thorough and Compassionate Responses

Just as important as encouraging questions is making sure the answers we give are detailed, clear, and kind. Providing a quick response or going into overly technical details can create more confusion. It's essential to fully engage with the patient's question, adjusting the answer to match their understanding and emotional state.

A complete answer should address the question and show empathy and reassurance. For instance, when a patient asks about the risks of a kidney transplant, it's not enough to say, "There are risks involved, but we will monitor you closely." While that's true, it might leave the patient feeling anxious. A better response could be, "It's completely normal to be concerned about the risks of a transplant. There are risks, just like with any surgery, but rest assured, we will take every step to minimize those risks and ensure you are well taken care of throughout the process."

Moreover, checking for understanding is very important. Medical providers can ask if the patient needs further clarification or summarize key points to ensure they understand the information. After discussing the kidney transplant process, providers might say, "Does that make sense? Is there anything I can explain in more detail?" This allows the patient to express any lingering confusion.

Providing thorough responses shows that providers genuinely care about the patient's well-being and are dedicated to giving them all the information they need to make informed decisions. When patients leave a consultation feeling satisfied with the answers they've received, they're more likely to trust the provider and the treatment plan. This trust is key to building a stronger relationship and enhancing patient outcomes.

A powerful historical example of the importance of encouraging patient questions and providing thorough responses can be found in the story of Dr. Paul Farmer, a renowned physician and anthropologist who co-founded PIH, an organization dedicated to providing health care to impoverished communities worldwide.

Dr. Farmer's work in Haiti beautifully showcases how meaningful patient communication can enhance health outcomes. He firmly believed in the importance of engaging with patients in a way that respected their voices and perspectives. For him, health care went beyond just delivering medical treatment; it was about building personal connections and ensuring patients grasped their health and treatment choices.

In the rural areas of Haiti, many patients had limited formal education, which made understanding complex medical concepts quite challenging for them. Rather than dismissing their inquiries or oversimplifying explanations, Dr. Farmer took the time to thoroughly clarify ideas, connecting with patients at their level of understanding. For instance, when working with tuberculosis patients, he would patiently explain how the disease spreads, stress the importance of completing the entire treatment course, and discuss the risks associated with stopping treatment prematurely. He made sure his patients understood what their treatment involved and why it mattered. A key part of Dr. Farmer's approach was his belief in engaging patients as active participants in their care. He welcomed questions, no matter how small they seemed, and reassured them that their concerns were significant. For example, if a patient wondered why they needed to take a pill every day or worried about side effects, Dr. Farmer would take those questions to heart, providing clear answers and addressing any fears. He recognized that patients are more likely to adhere to treatment and care instructions when they feel heard.

One remarkable story features a Haitian woman named Marie, who faced a diagnosis of tuberculosis. Her treatment plan involved a complicated array of medications, and at first, she felt unsure about following it due to her lack of understanding regarding the purpose of each medication and the importance of sticking to the regimen. Dr. Farmer noticed her hesitation and took the time to sit down with Marie, explaining the science behind her illness and how each medication contributed to her recovery. He encouraged her to ask questions and ensured she felt empowered with the knowledge necessary to manage her health. By creating a space for open dialogue and providing clear answers, he helped her grasp her condition and established a trusting relationship. Marie adhered to the treatment plan and ultimately made a full recovery.

Dr. Farmer's method of communicating with patients not only enhanced health outcomes but also transformed how patients perceived their roles within the health care system. His knack for fostering questions and delivering comprehensive, compassionate explanations cultivated a partnership between him and his patients. This collaborative approach was crucial to the success of his efforts in Haiti and other underserved communities worldwide [3, 12, 18].

As health care providers, we must understand how much communication influences the patient experience. When we encourage patients to ask questions—no matter how small—we create a welcoming environment where they can share their concerns, express their feelings, and take an active role in their health care. Using techniques that promote open conversation, like open-ended questions and a friendly atmosphere, can help patients feel more involved and empowered in their care.

## Conclusion

In conclusion, effective communication in health care is foundational to delivering compassionate and patient-centered care. The chapter highlights the profound impact of active listening, empathy, and reflective listening on building trust and improving patient outcomes. By mastering the art of asking thoughtful questions and understanding nonverbal cues, health care providers can foster deeper connections with their patients, ensuring they feel heard, understood, and empowered. Simplifying complex medical information and encouraging patients to ask questions further strengthens the doctor-patient relationship, enhancing engagement and collaboration in care decisions. Ultimately, the chapter reinforces that communication is about transferring information and creating meaningful, supportive relationships that help patients navigate their health care journey with confidence and dignity.

**Take-Home Points**

- **Active listening and empathy** are essential for building trust and improving outcomes in any professional relationship.
- **Reflective listening** helps people feel understood and fosters stronger connections.
- **Asking open-ended and probing questions** encourages deeper engagement and clearer understanding in conversations.
- **Nonverbal cues** (such as body language and tone) provide crucial insights into emotions and thoughts in all interactions.
- **Simplifying complex information** and encouraging questions help increase understanding and empower decision-making in any setting.

## References

1. Bliss M. William Osler: a life in medicine. Oxford: Oxford University Press; 2007.
2. Burlingame M. Abraham Lincoln: a life. Baltimore: Johns Hopkins University Press; 2023.
3. Farmer P. Pathologies of power: health, human rights, and the new war on the poor. Berkeley: University of California Press; 2004.
4. Freud S. The interpretation of dreams: the complete and definitive text. New York: Basic Books; 2010.
5. Goleman D. Social intelligence: the new science of human relationships. New York: Bantam; 2007.
6. Goodwin DK. Team of rivals: the political genius of Abraham Lincoln. New York: Simon & Schuster; 2006.
7. Hamilton A. Exploring the dangerous trades. New York: Lugubrious; 2017.
8. Josef Breuer SF. Studies on hysteria, Basic Books classics. New York: Basic Books; 2000.
9. Marshall BJ, Warren JR. Unidentified curved bacilli in the stomach of patients with gastritis and peptic ulceration. Lancet. 1984;1(8390):1311–5. https://doi.org/10.1016/s0140-6736(84)91816-6.
10. Ofri D. What patients say, what doctors hear. Boston: Beacon Press; 2017.
11. Oshinsky D. Polio: an American story. Oxford: Oxford University Press; 2005.
12. Paul Farmer AK, Kim JY. Reimagining global health: an introduction. Berkeley: University of California Press; 2013.
13. Phillips D. Lincoln on leadership: executive strategies for tough times. Marion: Donald T Phillips & Associates; 2013.
14. Remen RN. Kitchen table wisdom: stories that heal. New York: Riverhead Books; 2006.
15. Riedel S. Edward Jenner and the history of smallpox and vaccination. Proc (Bayl Univ Med Cent). 2005;18(1):21–5. https://doi.org/10.1080/08998280.2005.11928028.
16. Rogers N. Polio wars: Sister Kenny and the Golden Age of American medicine. Oxford: Oxford University Press; 2013.
17. Sicherman B. Alice Hamilton: a LIFE IN LETTERS. Champaign: University of Illinois Press; 2003.
18. Tracy Kidder PM. Mountains beyond mountains: the quest of Dr Paul Farmer, a man who would cure the world. New York: Random House Audio; 2003.
19. Verghese A. Culture shock—patient as icon, icon as patient. N Engl J Med. 2008;359(26):2748–51. https://doi.org/10.1056/NEJMp0807461.

# 6 Shared Decision-Making

In a busy city hospital, Dr. Emily Stone found herself at a crucial moment with her patient, Tom, a middle-aged man who had just been diagnosed with type 2 diabetes. The room buzzed with the sound of medical equipment. Yet, the atmosphere was thick with tension as Tom struggled to come to terms with his new situation, his expression showing the shock and bewilderment that often accompanies a sudden chronic illness diagnosis.

Dr. Stone, recognized for her careful approach and genuine compassion, understood her interaction with Tom could greatly influence his health results. "Tom," she said softly, "you have some key decisions ahead regarding diabetes management. I'm here to provide more than just medical advice; I want to help and support you as you navigate these choices." As she talked, she outlined the treatment options, explaining how diet, medication, and lifestyle changes could impact his long-term health. Tom listened, and his initial nervousness gradually turned into curiosity. "So, how do we decide what's best for me?" he inquired, appearing a bit overwhelmed.

Dr. Stone offered a warm smile, recognizing the importance of collaboration in his care. "Let's discuss what matters most to you," she encouraged. "Is it managing side effects, keeping up with your current lifestyle, or perhaps something different?" This straightforward question changed the tone of the conversation, allowing Tom to engage more actively. He shared his worries about missing out on family meals and the burden of medication expenses. Dr. Stone listened carefully, validating his concerns and tailoring her suggestions to fit his values and priorities in life.

Together, they developed a tailored management plan that effectively controlled Tom's diabetes while respecting his wish for a lifestyle with minimal interruptions. Dr. Stone ensured Tom grasped every part of the plan, including how the medications worked and when to check his blood glucose. This teamwork not only provided Tom with the tools he needed to manage his diabetes but also fostered a feeling of control and collaboration. When he left the office that day, he took a treatment plan and a refreshed confidence in his ability to shape his health outcomes.


F. Aziz, *The Healing Art of Connecting with Patients*,
https://doi.org/10.1007/978-3-032-03624-7_6

Dr. Stone observed him as he walked away, filled with a deep satisfaction. She realized that involving patients like Tom in shared decision-making not only customized their medical treatments but also fostered trust and encouraged her patients to participate in their care actively. This transformed the doctor-patient relationship into a genuine partnership. She thought this is the kind of modern health care we should aim for, where every patient feels appreciated, understood, and engaged in their path to wellness.

Let's delve into history to understand the significance of collaborative decision-making. Back in 1975, during a spring evening, a 21-year-old woman named Karen Ann Quinlan was taken to the hospital after falling into a coma due to a mix of alcohol and sedatives. As a result, she experienced significant brain damage and remained in a persistent vegetative state. This situation presented a heartbreaking truth to her parents, Joseph and Julia Quinlan: their daughter was being sustained on a ventilator with no chances of improvement.

Karen's parents wanted her to pass away peacefully, but the doctors declined to remove life support, citing ethical concerns despite Karen's slim chance of recovery. The family felt devastated and helpless, excluded from decisions about their daughter's fate. The Quinlans embarked on a significant legal fight questioning the conventional, paternalistic approach to medical decision-making. They presented their case to the New Jersey Supreme Court, which decided in their favor in 1976, supporting their ability to withdraw Karen from life support. This pivotal ruling marked the first recognition that patients and families should play a role in end-of-life care choices, a notable shift from the belief that doctors exclusively determined such decisions.

Karen continued to breathe independently after the ventilator was removed, living in a vegetative state for nearly a decade until her passing in 1985. Her situation had a lasting impact on medical ethics, shaping modern concepts of patient autonomy, informed consent, and shared decision-making. The Quinlan case marked a pivotal moment, emphasizing that medical knowledge, while important, must be complemented by the perspectives of the patient and their family. It highlighted the vital reality that health care decisions go beyond clinical matters, reflecting personal values, beliefs, and the sanctity of human life [25, 38].

This story reminds us why SDM is more than a modern approach; it is a moral and ethical necessity, ensuring every patient's voice is heard and respected, even when facing life's most difficult crossroads.

## Introduction to Shared Decision-Making (SDM)

The relationship between patients and medical providers has undergone a profound transformation in the contemporary health care environment. No longer are patients passive recipients of care; they are now active participants in their health care journey. This shift has been fueled by the increasing availability of medical information, a greater emphasis on patient rights, and the recognition that health care is most effective when personalized and patient-centered.

SDM lies at the heart of this transformation. It is a collaborative process in which health care providers and patients work together to make decisions that best suit the patient's needs, preferences, and values. This approach recognizes that while medical providers bring essential expertise, patients get their unique perspectives and lived experiences.

Let's consider a hypothetical scenario. Picture a young woman named Maria who has been diagnosed with a chronic autoimmune illness. Despite numerous visits to the doctor over the years, her condition has worsened. Now, she is confronted with a crucial choice: should she opt for a risky surgery that could bring long-term advantages or stick with conservative treatment that guarantees a more modest outcome?

Anxious but hopeful, Maria sits across from her doctor, Dr. Lewis, who explains the pros and cons of each option in clinical terms. Initially, the conversation feels one-sided, with Dr. Lewis detailing statistical success rates and possible complications. Maria listens, but her mind swirls with emotions—her fear of the unknown, her desire to live an active life, and the impact her choice will have on her family.

Sensing Maria's hesitation, Dr. Lewis shifts the conversation. Instead of continuing with data and probabilities, he asks, "*Maria, what matters most to you in this decision? What are your concerns and priorities?*"

Suddenly, the dynamic changes. Maria feels seen, her voice valued. She expresses her fear of being unable to care for her children if the surgery goes wrong, but also her longing to regain the energy to live fully again. Dr. Lewis listens intently, acknowledging the medical facts and Maria's unique perspective. Together, they explore different paths, discussing what is medically possible and what aligns with Maria's life goals and values.

This is the essence of SDM—an approach where medical providers and patients collaborate to find a solution not only clinically sound but also aligns with the patient's needs and personal values. SDM is not just about presenting choices; it's about creating a meaningful dialogue where both parties contribute to the final decision.

The doctor-patient relationship, often one of the most meaningful human interactions, is central to medicine. Trust, mutual respect, and a shared goal of improving the patient's health define this relationship. As the health care landscape continues to evolve with a stronger focus on patient rights and personalization, fostering this relationship through SDM is critical.

## Historical Perspective: The Evolution of Doctor-Patient Relationships

The doctor-patient relationship is a cornerstone of medical practice, shaping how care is delivered and received. Its evolution reflects broader changes in society and medical ethics. As medical knowledge and societal values have progressed, so have the models describing how medical providers and patients interact. In 1956, the famous psychiatrists Thomas Szasz and Marc Hollender introduced three basic

**Table 6.1** Models of patient-doctor relationships

| Model name | Description | Historical context | Modern perspective/ application |
|---|---|---|---|
| Active-passive model | The traditional paternalistic approach involves the health care provider making decisions primarily independently, with little input from the patient. | Prominent in the early twentieth century, it was primarily utilized in emergency or critical care situations where swift decisions were essential | This is still relevant when patients can't make decisions for themselves (like when they're unconscious), with choices being made ethically to prioritize the patient's best interests |
| Guidance-cooperation model | The medical provider offers guidance, and the patient is encouraged to participate in the process while following those recommendations | This was brought to light in the mid-twentieth century as medical science progressed and patients took more control over their health | It is helpful in scenarios where straightforward medical advice is needed while allowing for some patient involvement, mainly when complicated choices aren't necessary |
| Mutual participation model | The most advanced approach focuses on shared decision-making, highlighting the importance of patient autonomy and their involvement in care choices | It evolved from the civil rights and patient rights movements, highlighting the significance of holistic care and the need for informed consent | Regarded as the gold standard, especially for handling chronic conditions and in patient-centered care settings, it encourages meaningful collaborative conversations |

models that have become foundational in medical education and practice [43]. These models—the Active-Passive, Guidance-Cooperation, and Mutual Participation—represent distinct health care decision-making approaches and highlight the shift toward more patient-centered care over time (Table 6.1).

## The Active-Passive Model

The Active-Passive Model was dominant in the early twentieth century when medical paternalism was the norm. Medical providers were viewed as authoritative figures whose knowledge and expertise were beyond question. Patients were expected to comply without input or consent. Informed consent—a fundamental principle in modern medicine—was not yet established. Nowhere is the peril of this one-sided approach more tragically illustrated than in the treatment of US President James A. Garfield after an assassination attempt in 1881.

On July 2, 1881, President Garfield was shot twice by a disgruntled office seeker, Charles J. Guiteau, at the Baltimore and Potomac train station in Washington, DC. Although one bullet grazed his arm, the other lodged deep in his back. It missed vital organs and major arteries—by today's standards, a non-fatal injury. Medical historians widely agree that, with appropriate care, Garfield likely would have survived. However, he became a victim not of the assassin's bullet but of the medical practices dictated by the paternalistic Active-Passive Model.

From the moment Garfield was wounded, his care was led by Dr. D. Willard Bliss, a well-known physician who took complete control over the President's treatment. Operating under the belief that a physician's judgment was supreme, Bliss dismissed input from other doctors and even ignored Garfield's discomfort and expressions of pain. The President, the most powerful man in the country, was rendered powerless over his own body—a stark example of the Active-Passive Model in action.

Driven by the era's belief that locating and removing the bullet was paramount, Dr. Bliss began an aggressive and invasive search. He inserted his unwashed fingers and non-sterile instruments into the wound repeatedly. These examinations were carried out despite Garfield's suffering and without his informed consent—because, under the paternalistic model, consent was not considered necessary. The physician's knowledge was deemed superior to the patient's experience of pain or fear.

At the time, germ theory—pioneered by Louis Pasteur and Joseph Lister—was gaining acceptance in Europe, emphasizing the importance of antiseptic techniques. However, American doctors, including Bliss, largely rejected these ideas as unnecessary. Bliss believed his skill and experience alone were sufficient, a common mindset in the Active-Passive Era, where a physician's authority went unquestioned.

Garfield endured 80 days of unimaginable suffering. His condition deteriorated as repeated probing introduced infections, leading to sepsis and the formation of pus-filled abscesses along his spine. His once-robust frame withered away as he became emaciated. He developed a severe fever, chills, and constant pain, all while being subjected to experimental feeding techniques, including nutrient enemas—a desperate attempt to sustain him when he could no longer eat.

Throughout this ordeal, Garfield's voice was silenced. He had no role in his treatment decisions. His fate rested entirely in Bliss's hands. Even as his condition worsened and other physicians voiced concerns, Bliss maintained his position as the final authority. The notion Garfield—or his family—might participate in medical decisions was inconceivable within the Active-Passive framework. On September 19, 1881, Garfield succumbed to infection, not the bullet. An autopsy revealed the bullet had lodged harmlessly near his spine and could have remained there indefinitely without causing death. The real cause was the infection introduced by the repeated probing and lack of sterile care—a lethal consequence of Bliss's unchecked authority and the pervasive paternalism of the time.

Garfield's passing was a distressing event that captured the nation's attention, with his prolonged suffering making headlines. Beyond its political impact, his death prompted deep contemplation within the medical field. It was a poignant reminder of the importance of combining medical expertise with scientific evidence and patient involvement.

Although it would take decades for the medical profession to fully embrace patient autonomy and informed consent, Garfield's suffering planted seeds of doubt about the infallibility of the physician; his case highlighted the dangers of absolute medical authority and the perils of ignoring emerging scientific advancements, such as antiseptic techniques. Over time, it contributed to the gradual erosion of the Active-Passive Model as the universal standard of care [32].

The Active-Passive Model still finds its place today—mainly when patients are unconscious or unable to make decisions. Yet the lesson from Garfield's suffering endures: When the patient's voice is silenced, and the physician's authority is unchecked, the risk of harm increases.

As Dr. Eric Cassell reminds us, "The purpose of medical ethics is to ensure that the physician acts in the best interest of the patient, even when the patient cannot make decisions" [6]. Garfield's story reminds us that the physician's best intentions must always be tempered by humility, science, and respect for the patient's humanity.

## The Guidance-Cooperation Model

The Guidance-Cooperation Model represents a more balanced and collaborative approach to the doctor-patient relationship, sitting between the paternalistic Active-Passive Model and the modern emphasis on shared decision-making. In this model, the medical provider takes on the role of an expert advisor, offering guidance based on their medical knowledge and clinical experience. The patient is encouraged to participate by asking questions and expressing concerns, but they are ultimately expected to comply with the treatment plan. Decision-making authority still primarily rests with the provider, especially when the patient lacks the medical understanding to make informed choices.

Imagine a scenario where a person has recently been diagnosed with type 2 diabetes. The doctor discusses the significance of managing blood glucose levels by following a balanced diet, engaging in physical activity, and taking prescribed medication. The individual might have questions about the potential side effects of the medication or find it challenging to stick to a strict diet. While the patient's concerns are considered, the doctor's advice is crucial in shaping the treatment strategy. The patient's responsibility is to collaborate with the suggested treatment plan, having faith in the doctor's expertise to attain optimal health results. This dynamic showcases a partnership where the patient trusts the doctor's knowledge while participating in the health care journey.

In the 1940s, the introduction of penicillin and other antibiotics marked a significant shift in medical practice. Patients were guided by physicians on the proper use of these revolutionary drugs, emphasizing the importance of completing the entire course for effectiveness. This era highlighted the Guidance-Cooperation Model, acknowledging the crucial role of patient adherence in successful treatment outcomes.

The Guidance-Cooperation Model gained prominence during the mid-twentieth century, as advancements in medical science, pharmaceuticals, and diagnostic tools empowered physicians to offer more precise treatments. Patients had more influence over their care, but the doctor's authority remained central. Compliance with prescribed treatments was emphasized, particularly in chronic disease management.

Today, this model remains relevant in cases where patients require structured medical guidance but may lack the capacity, knowledge, or desire to make complex health care decisions. Conditions such as diabetes, hypertension, and post-surgical recovery often require patients to adhere closely to medical instructions. In these contexts, the physician's expertise is critical, while the patient's cooperation ensures successful outcomes.

Nonetheless, there remain scenarios where patients—due to illness, complexity of treatment, or personal preference—rely heavily on their doctor's guidance. The Guidance-Cooperation Model reminds health care providers that while expert knowledge is invaluable, fostering patient understanding and encouraging cooperation leads to better adherence and improved health outcomes.

## The Mutual Participation Model

The rise of the Mutual Participation Model reflects broader social movements and legal developments in the mid-to-late twentieth century that fundamentally reshaped the doctor-patient relationship. These historical milestones emphasized patient autonomy, informed consent, and the right to participate in medical decisions, challenging the previously entrenched paternalistic approach.

One of the most influential cases in establishing informed consent as a legal and ethical standard in medicine was Canterbury v. Spence. This landmark ruling emerged from the experience of Jerry Canterbury, a 19-year-old patient who underwent spinal surgery without being adequately informed of the risks. The operation, performed by Dr. William Spence, resulted in paralysis due to an undisclosed complication.

Canterbury's lawsuit argued that patients had the right to know the risks associated with any medical procedure before consenting to it. The US Court of Appeals for the District of Columbia ruled in his favor, establishing that physicians must disclose information that a reasonable person would find necessary to make an informed decision. The ruling effectively shifted the balance of power in the doctor-patient relationship, acknowledging patients are not passive recipients but active decision-makers in their health care [5].

The Canterbury decision became a cornerstone of the Mutual Participation Model, embedding informed consent into modern medical ethics and reinforcing that patients have the right to be partners in their care.

The Tuskegee Syphilis Study is a significant and troubling chapter in American medical history, highlighting a serious breach of trust, especially when contrasted with important legal milestones like the Canterbury v. Spence ruling, which promoted patient rights through informed consent. This troubling study, initiated by the US Public Health Service in 1932, is a clear example of a major ethical failure. It falsely promised free health care to African American men in Macon County,

Alabama, while misleading them about their condition and depriving them of essential treatment.

In the 1940s, when penicillin was discovered as a clear cure for syphilis, many men were unfortunately left to endure the painful effects of their illness. This study went on for a heartbreaking 40 years, during which these individuals faced unimaginable challenges as their health declined due to lack of treatment. The impact was severe: numerous men lost their lives, while others dealt with lasting issues like blindness, mental health struggles, and ongoing pain. Additionally, the disease quietly affected their families, spreading to partners and children, creating a cycle of suffering that reached far beyond the original participants.

Uncovering this troubling chapter in 1972 deeply affected the nation's conscience and sparked widespread outrage. The significant ethical violations led to an urgent national dialogue about the importance of trust and moral responsibility in health care. In response to this collective shock, the National Research Act of 1974 created institutional review boards to monitor medical research and enforce strict informed consent regulations. These initiatives were designed to rebuild the trust that had been broken between the medical community and the public, ensuring such ethical missteps would not happen again.

The impact of Tuskegee is lasting, creating a deep-seated distrust that resonates through generations, especially in the African American community. It serves as a poignant reminder of the dangers of treating patients as mere subjects instead of recognizing them as valuable individuals worthy of honesty, respect, and care. This historical violation of ethical responsibility highlights the necessity for vigilance and integrity in medical practice, ensuring patient autonomy is prioritized over scientific curiosity [4, 23].

During the 1960s and 1970s, the Women's Health Movement arose alongside feminist activism, advocating for women's autonomy over their bodies and reproductive health decisions. Historically, women's concerns were often dismissed by male physicians, and reproductive health procedures, such as sterilizations or hysterectomies, were sometimes performed without their full consent.

Publications like *Our Bodies, Ourselves* (1971) empowered women by providing accessible, non-paternalistic medical information, enabling them to engage more actively in health care decisions. The movement also led to landmark reproductive rights cases, such as Roe v. Wade (1973), which affirmed a woman's right to make autonomous decisions regarding pregnancy [3].

The Women's Health Movement, which gained momentum in the latter part of the twentieth century, marked a substantial change in health care perspectives, especially highlighting women's roles as engaged partners in their medical care. This movement played a key role in promoting the Mutual Participation Model, viewing patients, particularly women, as essential collaborators in the decision-making process rather than mere recipients of care. This transformation challenged conventional dynamics where doctors were the only decision-makers, creating a space where patients' voices and preferences were acknowledged and appreciated.

During the 1980s and 1990s, the HIV/AIDS crisis emerged as a significant force for promoting patient autonomy and collaborative health care. Encountering widespread discrimination, stigma, and a lack of adequate government response, those impacted by HIV/AIDS rose, turning their struggles into a powerful movement for change. Groups like ACT UP and the AIDS Coalition to Unleash Power became key players, representing the voices and needs of the community. These activists were not just fighting for their survival; they insisted on being heard and included in the discussions that shaped their futures.

Patients living with HIV/AIDS have become powerful advocates, not just receiving the benefits of medical research but actively shaping it as well. They bravely challenged the norms, standing up to doctors, pharmaceutical companies, and government agencies. Their push for faster drug approvals and the creation of more compassionate, patient-centered research protocols has led to a remarkable shift in health care. They asserted their right to be informed and to make independent choices about experimental treatments, establishing new benchmarks for patient involvement and empowerment in their health management. This movement has not only transformed policies but also significantly changed how patients engage with the health care system, ensuring their voices and choices are at the forefront of the health care conversation [18, 40, 42].

These movements redefined the patient's role, transforming patients from passive recipients into informed advocates—a defining characteristic of the Mutual Participation Model.

## The Power and Advantages of Shared Decision-Making

SDM is not just a method; it is a philosophy that redefines the relationship between health care providers and patients. By fostering a collaborative environment, SDM empowers patients, enhances the quality of care, and strengthens the clinician-patient bond. This approach has profound implications, leading to increased satisfaction, better health outcomes, and more resilient health care systems.

### Patient Satisfaction

One of the most profound impacts of SDM in health care is the increase in patient satisfaction. In traditional models, patients often felt like passive recipients, with critical decisions made on their behalf without much input. SDM changes this dynamic entirely, placing patients at the center of their health care journey. This shift empowers patients to take an active role in their care, enhancing their engagement and overall health care experience. As the renowned Dr. Albert Schweitzer, who was a theologian, organist, musicologist, writer, humanitarian, philosopher, and physician, wisely stated, "Patients require rest, nourishment, fresh air, and physical activity—today, they also need trust, teamwork, and the opportunity to make informed decisions regarding their care" [39].

Patients involved in their health care decisions feel more respected, valued, and heard. The essence of SDM is not just about giving patients the ability to express their preferences, but recognizing them as equal partners in the decision-making process. When patients are empowered to share their goals, ask questions, and voice concerns, it fosters collaboration and partnership between the patient and medical provider. This involvement cultivates a more profound sense of ownership over treatment decisions, often resulting in greater adherence to prescribed care plans. As Dr. Angela Coulter, a health policy analyst and researcher from the UK who focuses on patient and public engagement, beautifully put it, "Nothing about me without me"—this principle highlights how crucial it is for patients to be part of the decision-making process [8].

Before the 1990s, breast cancer treatment decisions were often made without much input from patients. Many women diagnosed with breast cancer were quickly scheduled for radical mastectomies. This approach, advocated by Dr. William Halsted in the early twentieth century, became the norm for many years. Alternative, less invasive treatments like lumpectomy with radiation were not commonly discussed with patients. Physicians were typically viewed as the ultimate authority, and patients were expected to follow their recommendations without question.

In the 1990s, there was a significant movement led by breast cancer survivors and advocates, resulting in the emergence of organizations such as Breast Cancer Action and the National Breast Cancer Coalition (NBCC). These groups pushed for transparency, patient education, and inclusion in treatment decisions. Women questioned the standard surgical practices, advocating for less invasive options that considered both survival rates and quality of life.

A notable catalyst was the case of Rose Kushner, a journalist diagnosed with breast cancer in 1974. She rejected the traditional approach, which often involved biopsy and radical mastectomy in a single operation without consulting the patient. Kushner insisted on exploring alternative treatments and ultimately opted for a lumpectomy with radiation. Her outspoken advocacy and book, *Breast Cancer: A Personal History and Investigative Report* (1975), empowered countless women to question their doctors and demand involvement in their care decisions. Her efforts contributed to shifting the standard of care, promoting informed choice, and laying the groundwork for SDM in breast cancer treatment [28, 30].

Patient advocacy has led to an increase in SDM in breast cancer care. Women are now actively involved in discussions about surgical options, reconstruction, chemotherapy, and radiation. This collaborative approach has enhanced patient satisfaction by empowering women to shape their treatment paths. This patient-centered care model, emphasizing the value of SDM, is now being adopted across various health care specialties.

A highly impactful example of how SDM can enhance patient satisfaction is the transformation of childbirth practices from the 1950s to today. In the mid-twentieth century, childbirth in Western hospitals was often highly medicalized and paternalistic, with women having limited information and choices in their labor and delivery. Routine interventions, such as sedation, forceps deliveries, and episiotomies, were commonly performed without consent. Fathers were usually excluded from the delivery room, and mothers were discouraged from questioning medical decisions, leaving them disoriented and disempowered after birth.

The 1960s and 1970s marked the emergence of the natural childbirth movement, championed by figures like Dr. Grantly Dick-Read, Fernand Lamaze, and Sheila Kitzinger, alongside feminist health advocates. These people advocated for women to take back control of their birth experiences, emphasizing education, informed consent, and patient choice. Women began creating birth plans, requesting to be awake during delivery, and insisting on their partners' presence during labor. Midwives and doulas reemerged as patient advocates, assisting women in expressing their preferences and collaborating with health care providers. This shift toward SDM empowered women to discuss pain management, delivery methods, and post-birth preferences, leading to improved patient satisfaction [11, 13, 26].

The integration of SDM into maternity care significantly increased patient satisfaction levels. Women reported feeling more in control, respected, and emotionally supported, even in cases requiring medical intervention. The childbirth revolution illustrates how including patients in significant experiences enhances their sense of agency, trust in their health care team, and overall contentment.

Looking back on my journey as a transplant nephrologist, one experience stands out and beautifully highlights the significance of SDM in health care. It was about a middle-aged man, a passionate mountain biker, who received a life-changing diagnosis of end-stage kidney disease. His transformation from feeling anxious to actively engaging in his treatment decisions truly emphasizes the importance of considering patients' lifestyles and values in their medical care.

In our first consultation, we delved into more than just his medical history; we chatted about his love for biking, his family life, and the little joys in his day-to-day. This friendly exchange laid the groundwork for a partnership that transcended the usual patient-doctor relationship. As we investigated transplant options, including the differences between living and deceased donor organs, his interest blossomed as he gained a more precise understanding.

His main worry was the immunosuppressive drugs he would need to take after the transplant and how their side effects might affect his active lifestyle. To tackle this, we teamed up with a pharmacologist to customize the immunosuppressive plan, focusing on reducing its impact on his vibrant life. This effort was not only about achieving the best medical results but also about ensuring his treatment matched his identity and life aspirations.

Opting for a kidney from a living donor was his informed decision, motivated by the prospect of faster recovery and better long-term outcomes that would allow him to return to his biking trails more quickly. The moment he shared his achievement of returning to the trails after recovery remains one of the most rewarding of my professional life.

This experience has greatly influenced my perspective on medicine. It strengthened my dedication to viewing each patient not merely as someone receiving care but as an engaged partner in their health journey. SDM involves acknowledging patients as complete individuals and incorporating their values and preferences into clinical choices. This method improves the effectiveness of medical treatments and guarantees care is truly centered around the patient, leading to improved health outcomes.

## Medical Provider Fulfillment

For medical providers, SDM offers much more than just a method of patient care—it provides a profoundly fulfilling professional experience. In an SDM framework, the medical providers partner in the patient's journey, aligning treatment plans with the patient's values, preferences, and life circumstances. This collaborative approach leads to more personalized care and enhances the patient-provider relationship, often cited as one of the most rewarding aspects of medical practice. As Sir William Osler, one of the founders of modern medicine, once said, "Medicine is a science of uncertainty and an art of probability" [35]. SDM allows clinicians to navigate this uncertainty by incorporating the patient's unique perspectives, ultimately leading to more meaningful and patient-centered care.

When medical providers engage in SDM, they experience the satisfaction of providing care that genuinely resonates with their patients. Instead of merely dictating treatment plans, they actively involve patients in decision-making, ensuring the course of action aligns with the patient's goals and values. This approach reduces the likelihood of conflicts, misunderstandings, and dissatisfaction, common sources of stress and burnout among health care providers. By fostering a more profound connection with their patients, medical providers often find their work more rewarding, as they see firsthand how their care positively impacts patient satisfaction and overall health outcomes.

When medical providers engage in SDM, they not only share the responsibility of decision-making with patients but also create a more balanced and fulfilling practice. By encouraging patients to participate in their health care decisions actively, medical providers can reduce the emotional burden of making unilateral choices, particularly in complex or ethically challenging cases. The process of SDM fosters open communication, mutual respect, and trust, all of which contribute to a more positive work environment. As Dr. Michael Balint, a renowned psychoanalyst and physician, once noted, "The most frequently used drug in general practice is the doctor themselves" [1]. SDM helps medical providers maintain their well-being by focusing on relationships rather than transactional care, which can mitigate the isolation and emotional toll that leads to burnout.

A historical example that underscores the importance of aligning care with patient values can be traced back to the early twentieth century with the release of the Flexner Report in 1910. This report, commissioned by the Carnegie Foundation, revolutionized medical education in the United States and Canada by standardizing practices and promoting scientific rigor [16]. However, it also had unintended consequences. The intense focus on scientific expertise often led to a depersonalization of care, where the human aspects of medicine were sidelined. Medical providers, trained to prioritize clinical outcomes, often overlook patient preferences and values, contributing to patient dissatisfaction and clinician disillusionment.

In response to this shift, medical thinkers in the mid-twentieth century advocated for a more holistic, patient-centered approach to care. SDM embodies this principle by ensuring patient care is personalized and aligned with their unique circumstances. Medical providers who practice SDM often find greater professional satisfaction, as they can reconnect with the humanistic roots of medicine, providing care that honors both scientific excellence and individual patient needs.

By adopting SDM, medical providers can significantly reduce the emotional burden associated with patient care. When they witness the positive impact of their efforts, from improved patient contentment to better health outcomes, medical providers experience a renewed sense of purpose and fulfillment in their roles. This can be a powerful antidote to burnout, as it reinforces the intrinsic rewards of practicing medicine. A study published in the Journal of the American Medical Association found that medical providers who engaged in SDM reported higher job satisfaction and lower rates of burnout, primarily because they felt more connected to their patients and their professional mission [41].

In short, SDM not only enhances the patient experience but also offers medical providers a more fulfilling and sustainable way to practice medicine. By aligning treatment with patient values and reducing the risk of conflict, SDM fosters a more rewarding professional environment. In an era where medical providers' burnout is at an all-time high, the collaborative, patient-centered approach of SDM provides a pathway to a more balanced and meaningful practice.

During my internal medicine residency, I learned the critical importance of SDM in enhancing patient care and preventing physician burnout. Managing a middle-aged woman with chronic heart failure, I saw firsthand how previous negative experiences had led her to distrust the health care system. By engaging her through SDM, I sought to rebuild trust and involve her actively in her treatment planning.

We explored her values and life goals, and together, we crafted a treatment plan that prioritized her quality of life. This approach improved her treatment adherence and made the care process more rewarding for both of us. It underscored the importance of empathy, listening, and respect in health care. The positive outcome from this collaborative approach highlighted how SDM can significantly impact health outcomes and enhance physician satisfaction—crucial factors in mitigating burnout among health care providers.

In another instance during my nephrology training, I dealt with an elderly patient at a crucial decision-making point concerning his end-of-life care. This situation required delicate conversations about potential treatments and their impact on his quality of life. Through SDM, we involved him and his family in every discussion, aligning his medical care with his values and preferences. This process provided him with a sense of control and peace in his decisions and reinforced my resilience by connecting deeply with my patient's needs and values.

These experiences highlighted that SDM is beneficial for patients and vital for maintaining physicians' emotional and professional well-being. By fostering a collaborative environment, SDM helps reduce the emotional toll on physicians, combating burnout by ensuring the caregiving process is as fulfilling as it is curative. This dual benefit of SDM underscores its indispensable role in the health care system, reminding us of the powerful impact of true partnership between patients and health care providers on mutual well-being.

## Impact on Health Care Teams

SDM doesn't just benefit individual clinicians and patients; it profoundly impacts the broader health care team. When all team members—from nurses to allied health professionals—are actively involved in the SDM process, it creates a more cohesive, collaborative, and efficient work environment. By engaging the entire team in discussions about patient care, SDM promotes open communication, mutual respect, and a shared sense of responsibility, all of which contribute to higher-quality patient outcomes and increased job satisfaction for the health care team.

Incorporating SDM within a health care team means every member, from the medical provider to the dietitian or physical therapist, is encouraged to contribute their expertise and insights. This multidisciplinary approach provides a more comprehensive understanding of the patient's needs, leading to better care.

Historical evidence supports the positive effects of collaborative decision-making on health care teams. For example, the Veterans Health Administration (VHA), which serves millions of veterans across the United States, has long utilized team-based care models focusing on SDM. A study found the VHA's emphasis on interdisciplinary teamwork and SDM improved patient satisfaction and better health outcomes for veterans with chronic illnesses. By involving various team members in decision-making, the VHA created a more cohesive and efficient system of care that benefited both patients and providers [37].

When all health care team members are engaged in the SDM process, it fosters a culture of inclusion and mutual respect. Nurses, for instance, who often have the most frequent and direct contact with patients, play a crucial role in identifying patient concerns and helping translate complex medical information into understandable terms. Engaging nurses and other allied health professionals in SDM helps ensure the patient's voice is consistently heard throughout the care process. This inclusive approach can reduce communication errors, enhance patient safety, and improve health outcomes.

SDM can also help reduce conflicts within health care teams. In traditional hierarchical models of care, decision-making is often dominated by the medical providers, with other health care professionals having limited input. This can create tension, frustration, and misunderstandings within the team. However, by encouraging open dialogue and equal participation, SDM fosters an environment where each team member's expertise is valued and decisions are made collaboratively.

During my internal medicine residency, I encountered a touching case that significantly influenced my appreciation for SDM among health care teams, particularly in end-of-life care situations. The patient was a woman battling an advanced-stage cancer whose health had deteriorated despite our best efforts with aggressive treatments.

As her prognosis became increasingly grim, the medical team called for a multidisciplinary meeting to discuss her care. This meeting included oncologists, palliative care specialists, nurses, social workers, and her family members. Each participant brought a different perspective, all unified by ensuring the patient's remaining time was as comfortable and meaningful as possible.

The oncologists explained that continuing with aggressive treatment might not be very effective and could lead to more discomfort, with only a small chance of significantly extending her life. The palliative care team highlighted how crucial it is to focus on pain management and symptom relief to enhance her quality of life. Nurses shared their observations from daily care, mentioning the patient's growing fatigue and lesser tolerance for invasive procedures. Social workers talked about the emotional and psychological support that both the patient and her family would require during this period. During our conversation, the patient's family shared their cherished memories and insights about her desires, highlighting that she consistently valued the quality of life more than the length of treatment. Their contributions were essential in guiding the team's approach, ensuring the care plan reflected what mattered most to her.

Witnessing this collaborative decision-making process was a profound learning experience. It demonstrated how each team member's expertise contributed to a holistic understanding of the patient's needs. It facilitated a care plan that respected her wishes and provided her family with comfort and support.

This experience highlighted the significance of SDM in delivering compassionate, patient-centered care during end-of-life situations. It reminded me that alongside medical knowledge, empathy, effective communication, and honoring patient autonomy are crucial when dealing with terminal illnesses. As a resident, it strengthened my dedication to championing and implementing this approach in my future medical career, understanding collaborative care not only supports patients but also enhances the practice of medicine.

## Reducing Health Care Utilization

SDM has a significant potential to reduce health care utilization by preventing unnecessary procedures, hospitalizations, and interventions. This collaborative approach, where patients are fully informed about all treatment options, empowers them to make decisions that align with their preferences and values. As a result, patients are more likely to avoid treatments that might be costly, risky, or misaligned with their goals, which can reduce overall health care costs.

One fundamental way SDM reduces health care utilization is by helping patients avoid unnecessary interventions. For instance, a patient experiencing long-term lower back pain might be advised by one physician to undergo spinal surgery. However, during an SDM conversation, the medical provider discusses non-surgical alternatives, such as physical therapy, medication management, or lifestyle changes. The patient, who values minimal downtime and has concerns about the risks of surgery, opts for physical therapy. This decision avoids not only the inherent risks and recovery time of surgery but also reduces hospital costs and the potential for complications like infections or extended rehabilitation. As Dr. David Eddy, a pioneer in evidence-based medicine, once said, "Good medical practice is less about doing more, and more about doing what is appropriate" [14]. By aligning treatment plans with patient goals, SDM is critical in curbing unnecessary medical interventions.

Consider a 55-year-old patient diagnosed with osteoarthritis in their knee, contemplating elective knee replacement surgery. During an SDM consultation, the physician explains the potential risks of surgery, such as infections, long recovery periods, and the possibility of needing a second surgery in the future, along with alternative options, including pain management, weight loss, and physical therapy. The patient, who leads a relatively active life and prefers to avoid the long recovery period, decides against surgery in favor of a conservative management approach involving physical therapy and lifestyle changes. This decision reflects the patient's values and avoids the costly and resource-intensive surgery. In addition, it reduces the risk of complications that could lead to rehospitalization, thus minimizing health care utilization.

SDM can also reduce hospital readmissions and preventable hospitalizations. By ensuring patients fully understand their treatment plans and follow-up care, clinicians can help prevent complications that often lead to rehospitalization. For example, in the case of a patient with heart failure, SDM can be employed to discuss medication management, diet changes, and follow-up visits. This proactive, patient-centered approach ensures the patient is more engaged in their care, reducing the likelihood of complications that could result in readmission. As an SDM advocate, Dr. Victor Montori emphasizes, "Shared decision-making isn't just about deciding what's best—it's about making sure that the care the patient receives fits their lives and goals" [34].

In conclusion, SDM is a powerful tool in reducing health care utilization by fostering informed, patient-centered choices. By ensuring patients are fully aware of the risks, benefits, and alternatives to invasive procedures or hospitalizations, health care providers can help patients make decisions that not only improve their quality of life but also reduce unnecessary strain on health care resources.

## The 4-C Stepwise Model for Shared Decision-Making

Developing a strong connection with patients is essential for effective treatment outcomes. Allowing patients a say in their treatment plans makes them more likely to respect and adhere to the decisions made. To facilitate this, I propose the 4-C Stepwise Model, which can guide physicians in creating a collaborative and patient-centered approach (Fig. 6.1).

### Step 1: Develop a Culture of Trust

The initial step toward successful SDM is to cultivate a culture of trust. Trust is the cornerstone of every medical provider-patient relationship, and it should be fostered through ongoing, open, and compassionate actions from health care providers.

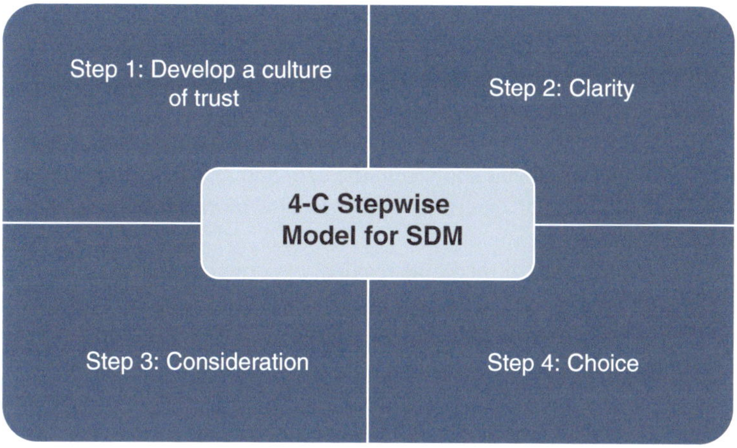


**Fig. 6.1** 4-C Stepwise Model for SDM

Stephen MR Covey, in his book *The Speed of Trust*, shares "Trust is the glue of life. It's the essential ingredient in effective communication. It's the foundational principle that holds all relationships" [9]. This perspective is critical in health care, where the medical provider-patient relationship can significantly affect treatment outcomes. Trust isn't something that comes automatically; it needs to be nurtured and sustained through actions that show integrity, clarity, and sincere care for the patient's well-being.

A culture of trust is essential for effective SDM in health care environments. Trust grows through consistent, open, and caring interactions between health care providers and patients, creating a space where communication and respect thrive. This strong foundation allows patients to feel comfortable expressing their concerns, asking questions, and actively participating in their treatment plans. When patients trust their health care providers, they are more likely to have meaningful conversations about their health options and stick to their treatment plans. Additionally, a culture of trust boosts patient satisfaction and compliance while promoting more effective, patient-centered care. Building this culture of trust is an active process that requires a continuous commitment from all health care professionals to listen, respond, and engage with patients in ways that honor their values and preferences.

The evolution of a culture of trust in health care has been significantly shaped by the groundbreaking efforts of individuals such as Dr. Francis W Peabody. His early twentieth-century contributions have laid the groundwork for our appreciation of patient-centered care.

Peabody's insights at Harvard Medical School transformed medical education and practice by highlighting the importance of the personal bond between doctors and patients in delivering effective health care. In his memorable 1926 lecture, he pointed out the shortcomings of the existing medical education system, which often focused more on the intricacies of diseases than on the actual practice of medicine concerning patient care. He championed a kinder, more empathetic approach that considers each patient's unique situation, concerns, and hopes [36].

Integrating this historical context into fostering a culture of trust highlights that building trust is a continuous journey grounded in consistent and empathetic patient engagement. Health care providers should emphasize open communication, actively listen to patient concerns, and show genuine care and respect for their values. This approach improves patient outcomes and creates a more effective and rewarding health care environment.

Reflecting on my internal medicine resident experiences, one case illustrates the profound importance of trust in the medical provider-patient relationship, especially during critical moments of health care decisions. I had the opportunity to care for a middle-aged patient who received an unexpected diagnosis of an aggressive cancer. Understandably, this news left the patient feeling overwhelmed by the sudden wave of information regarding treatment options, possible side effects, and prognosis. To make matters more challenging, the patient also struggled with significant anxiety and a lack of trust in the health care system, stemming from an experience where he felt his concerns were overlooked.

From the very beginning, it was evident that building trust was just as important as any medical treatment. In our initial meetings, I dedicated myself to fostering a supportive atmosphere where patients felt at ease sharing their fears and asking questions. I ensured each session allowed plenty of time to discuss the medical details and delve into the patient's feelings and reactions to the information shared. This method involved listening, acknowledging the patient's feelings, and responding empathetically. For every medical topic we discussed, I provided straightforward explanations. I took the time to answer the patient's questions, ensuring he had a complete grasp of his condition and the rationale for each recommended treatment. I also prioritized conversations about not just the clinical benefits of the treatments but also how they would impact the patient's quality of life, which was an essential concern for them.

As we navigated through this process, I could see a gradual change in the patient's demeanor from one of apprehension to one of engagement. The patient began to feel more confident in making informed decisions about his treatment options, expressing appreciation for the transparency and sensitivity with which the information was presented. This growing trust helped formulate a treatment plan that aligned closely with the patient's values and ensured they remained committed to the prescribed course of treatment.

This experience highlighted how essential trust is in health care. It showed me that while the technical side of medicine is critical, it's equally vital to have interpersonal skills that nurture trust and understanding. By the end of this journey, the patient felt more empowered, and his kind feedback and successful treatment management strengthened my dedication to practicing medicine with empathy and integrity. This case significantly impacted how I approach patient care, reminding me that the foundation of SDM is the trust we cultivate with our patients.

## Step 2: Clarity

Clarity plays a vital role in SDM. When communication between medical providers and patients is clear, complex medical issues are easier to understand. When patients grasp their medical situation completely, they can make better-informed choices, resulting in improved outcomes and increased adherence to treatment plans.

In my experience, I've observed effective medical providers often rely on simple tools like paper, pens, or whiteboards to visually outline complex medical issues and their potential solutions. This method makes intricate medical information easier to grasp, helping patients understand their conditions and the different treatment options available to them. By simplifying complicated concepts into manageable parts, these tools enable patients to make informed choices about their health care, boosting understanding and involvement. Adding clarity involves two essential practices: active listening and inviting questions—both of which are explored in depth in the chapter on communication.

A significant event in medical history that emphasizes the importance of clear SDM took place when President Dwight D. Eisenhower experienced a myocardial infarction in 1955. This incident revolutionized cardiac care in the United States and emphasized the crucial role of effective communication among doctors, patients, and the public in making well-informed health care choices. Eisenhower's situation is a historical illustration of how openness and patient engagement can enhance results and establish fresh benchmarks in medical care.

On September 24, 1955, President Eisenhower had a serious myocardial infarction while on vacation in Denver, Colorado. People knew little about heart disease, and heart care was still new. Dr. Paul Dudley White, a leading expert in cardiology, and his medical team had to make tough decisions while keeping Eisenhower, his family, and the public informed. As the President, Eisenhower's health was not just a personal issue but a national one, so they had to find the right balance between medical privacy, openness, and making the best choices [10].

Eisenhower's treatment was notable for its focus on open communication between physician and patient. Dr. White broke new ground by including Eisenhower in discussions about his treatment plan, explaining his condition, risks, and lifestyle changes. Eisenhower played an active role in making decisions about his recovery and stress management, which extended his life by 14 years [29].

Beyond the urgent health issues, maintaining clear communication with the public was crucial in influencing the country's reaction. Inaccurate information regarding the President's well-being might have caused economic and political turmoil. Dr. White and the medical staff offered regular, fact-based reports to the media and the public. This high level of openness comforted the nation, lessened anxiety, and built stronger confidence in health care. Additionally, the incident sparked a nationwide dialogue on cardiovascular disease, promoting preventive actions like quitting smoking, improving diet, and managing stress.

Eisenhower's myocardial infarction and medical response transformed cardiac care in the United States, influencing the growth of preventative cardiology and the establishment of coronary care units in hospitals. This laid the groundwork for modern cardiac intensive care and boosted the American Heart Association's role in public health education. Eisenhower's case highlights how effective communication enhances shared decision-making. Dr. White's patient-centered approach, emphasizing active listening, patient questions, and clear explanations, empowers patients in their health care journey. It underscores the importance of patients understanding their conditions, engaging in discussions with health care providers, and participating in decision-making for better health outcomes and patient satisfaction.

## Step 3: Consideration

Once the patient fully grasps their medical situation, the next important step is to have a detailed conversation about all available treatment options. This stage is where patient involvement becomes crucial. It's the moment when the patient and health care provider work together closely to evaluate the different options, considering the risks and benefits, to arrive at a well-informed, balanced, and harmonious decision with the patient's values.

### The Importance of Presenting Options Clearly

In the consideration phase, medical providers must present all available treatment options in a clear and unbiased manner. This is not merely a recitation of medical facts but a dialogue that empowers the patient to understand the implications of each choice. As the adage goes, "An informed patient is an empowered patient." Empowerment in this context means patients are not just aware of their options but also understand them well enough to evaluate the potential outcomes and make decisions they can fully support.

In his book *How Doctors Think*, Dr. Jerome Groopman highlights that "patients and their families require time to explore their choices, think about what suits them best, and have discussions with their doctors and other trusted advisors" [19]. This points out how crucial it is for patients to have the opportunity to reflect on their options, converse with their loved ones, and make decisions that take their overall life situations into account.

### Navigating the Complexities of Risk and Benefit

A key part of this step is chatting about the risks and benefits of each treatment option. Every medical choice comes with uncertainties; the medical provider's job is to help the patient navigate these complexities. This reminds us that medical providers should present risks and benefits in a way that recognizes uncertainty while helping the patient understand the probabilities.

When discussing risks, it's crucial to ensure patients aren't overwhelmed by potential downsides, nor should they receive false reassurances. The aim is to provide a balanced perspective, allowing the patient to weigh these risks against the possible benefits, considering their values and health goals. As patients reflect on these factors, they should feel at ease asking questions to understand how different treatment options might affect their daily lives, long-term health, and overall well-being.

### Facilitating a Thoughtful Decision-Making Process

During this step, medical providers should encourage patients to participate actively in decision-making. This involves more than just presenting options; it's about engaging the patient in a thoughtful consideration of how each option fits into their life. Dr. Atul Gawande, in his book, *Being Mortal: Medicine and What Matters in the End*, discusses the importance of understanding what matters most to the patient, stating, "Our ultimate goal, after all, is not a good death but a good life to the very end" [17]. This perspective is crucial when helping patients make decisions that reflect their priorities and values.

For example, a treatment that offers a high likelihood of extending life but with significant side effects may be less desirable to a patient who values quality of life over longevity. Conversely, another patient might prioritize aggressive treatment to prolong life despite the risks. Understanding these individual preferences is key to helping patients make decisions they are comfortable with and committed to.

### The Role of the Clinician in Empowering the Patient

Medical providers are essential in helping patients feel empowered during the decision-making phase. This empowerment is about equipping patients with the information they need to make informed choices and instilling the confidence to select the path that best fits their personal goals. This sense of respect and teamwork flourishes when patients know their preferences and concerns are genuinely valued in decision-making.

Consideration is crucial in the SDM process, emphasizing a balanced, open, and patient-focused approach. It goes beyond merely discussing treatment options; it involves having a meaningful conversation with the patient that honors their values, preferences, and concerns. By offering a thorough explanation of the risks and benefits of each choice and inviting patients to ask questions and reflect on their decisions, clinicians help empower patients to make choices they can wholeheartedly support.

In 1982, Barney Clark, a retired dentist aged 61, was faced with a critical decision due to end-stage heart failure. With no donor heart available, he was allowed to receive the Jarvik-7, the first permanent artificial heart developed by Dr. Robert Jarvik and his team at the University of Utah. This groundbreaking medical intervention involved significant risks, including stroke, infection, and an uncertain quality of life. After extensive discussions with Dr. William DeVries and his family, Clark chose to proceed, driven by the goal of advancing medical science for future patients [12].

On December 2, 1982, Clark had the groundbreaking surgery and lived 112 days with the artificial heart. While the operation was a success, his recovery was challenging. He faced various complications, such as infections, speech difficulties, and strokes that left him weakened. Despite the difficulties, Clark stayed true to his choice, believing his journey would influence future artificial heart advancements.

His case triggered ethical discussions on patient distress and medical research, underscoring the significance of effective communication in crucial medical choices.

Clark's situation is a significant illustration of collaborative decision-making, with the patient and medical professionals joining forces to thoughtfully assess the advantages and drawbacks of a cutting-edge yet uncertain therapy. His choice went beyond just prolonging life and focused on matching medical decisions with his values and aspirations. This case highlights the significance of patient independence in exploring all possible choices before committing to a transformative medical decision. It also emphasizes that making informed, carefully considered choices, even in experimental medicine, demands openness, patient involvement, and consideration for individual values.

## Step 4: Choice

The last and most empowering part of the SDM process is when the patient makes an informed choice with the guidance of their medical provider's expertise. This decision results from a collaborative effort that combines the patient's values and preferences with the clinical insights from the health care team. This step is incredibly important—it marks the moment when the patient moves from being a passive recipient of care to an active participant in their health journey.

### The Significance of Informed Choice

In health care, making an informed choice goes beyond just picking a treatment option; it's about making sure the patient understands what their decision means. This includes knowing the benefits, risks, possible outcomes, and how their choice might affect their overall quality of life. Medical providers must provide all the necessary information in a way that is easy to understand and relevant to the patient.

As leadership expert John C. Maxwell wisely stated, "People buy into the leader before they buy into the vision," highlighting how crucial trust is in this process [31]. When patients trust their medical team and feel their thoughts and feelings have been genuinely acknowledged, they are much more likely to embrace a treatment plan. This trust is the cornerstone of making informed choices.

### Ownership and Responsibility

Ownership is an essential result of the SDM process. When patients participate in selecting their treatment, they develop a sense of responsibility for the results of that choice. This sense of ownership is empowering; it shifts the treatment plan from being merely prescribed by a medical provider to a decision made by the patient, grounded in their understanding and personal values. By involving patients in the decision-making process, medical providers honor the individuality of each patient, allowing them to choose a path that resonates with their circumstances and life goals.

### Empowerment Through Choice

Empowerment plays a crucial role in patient-centered care. When patients make informed choices, they're not just picking a treatment but taking charge of their health and exercising their autonomy. This sense of empowerment significantly impacts patient engagement and adherence to treatment. Patients in control of their health decisions are more inclined to stick to their treatment plans, adopt healthier habits, and actively manage their health. Dr. Victor Montori, a prominent supporter of minimally disruptive medicine, highlights this by stating, "Patients are not passive recipients of care; they are the true agents of their health" [33]. This viewpoint underscores that a medical provider's role is to support and inform patients, enabling them to make choices that reflect their values and goals.

### Enhancing Confidence and Commitment

The decision-making process is important for boosting a patient's confidence in managing their health. When patients participate actively in selecting their treatment, they tend to feel more dedicated to the plan and assured of their ability to stick with it. This sense of confidence is especially vital for managing chronic conditions, where following through with treatment and lifestyle changes over the long term is crucial for achieving the best results.

Additionally, making choices creates a partnership between the patient and the clinician. As patients take a more active role in their care, the clinician transitions from being a commanding figure to a supportive guide. This change enhances the therapeutic relationship, which has been shown to significantly contribute to patient satisfaction and positive health outcomes.

A significant historical illustration of the value of choice in SDM can be seen in the contributions of Dr. Elisabeth Kübler-Ross and the advocacy for patient autonomy in end-of-life care. Before the late twentieth century, individuals with terminal illnesses often had limited involvement in treatment decisions, as many doctors refrained from sharing prognosis details or continued aggressive treatments despite patient distress. Kübler-Ross, a Swiss-American psychiatrist, transformed the approach of health care providers toward dying patients, championing their entitlement to make well-informed decisions about their treatment [27].

Through extensive interviews with terminally ill patients, Kübler-Ross discovered that patients desired to participate in decisions regarding their end-of-life care. Many expressed a preference to forgo futile treatments, prioritize comfort measures, and maintain dignity in their final days instead of undergoing unnecessary medical interventions. Her research, featured in *On Death and Dying* (1969), introduced the well-known five stages of grief and initiated a global dialogue on patient rights and the importance of SDM in palliative care. Her advocacy contributed to the hospice movement, which stressed patient-centered care, effective pain management, and emotional support, ensuring terminally ill individuals could decide how they wanted to spend their last days [7].

A modern and powerful instance of the importance of choice in shared decision-making is Angelina Jolie's decision to have a preventive double mastectomy in 2013. Jolie, an actress and humanitarian, made this decision upon discovering she carried a BRCA1 gene mutation, significantly increasing her risk of breast cancer (87% lifetime risk) and ovarian cancer (50% lifetime risk). With a family history of cancer and facing a challenging decision about her future health, Jolie's case emphasizes how informed choice, patient empowerment, and shared decision-making are vital in preventive care.

Working closely with her medical team, genetic counselors, and surgeons, she evaluated all options, including enhanced surveillance, chemoprevention, and risk-reducing surgery. After weighing the risks and benefits, she opted for a prophylactic double mastectomy, followed by ovary removal (oophorectomy) to further reduce her cancer risk. Her decision, based on detailed medical consultations, genetic counseling, and personal values, was not taken lightly, highlighting the core elements of SDM.

Jolie shared her journey in a New York Times op-ed titled "My Medical Choice," aiming to raise awareness about genetic testing and empower women to make informed health decisions. By educating herself, consulting experts, and considering how each option fits into her life goals, she showed how choice in SDM empowers patients to take control of their health in a way that feels right for them. Her openness also raised public awareness about genetic testing for hereditary cancers, leading to a surge in BRCA testing worldwide, known as the "Angelina Jolie effect." Jolie's case serves as a powerful reminder that informed choice is the ultimate goal of SDM, ensuring patients are active participants in their medical decisions [15, 22].

## Bringing the 4-C Model of SDM Together

The 4-C Stepwise Model for SDM is vital in improving patient care and satisfaction. Let's look at a hypothetical situation with a patient named Jane, who has just been diagnosed with early-stage breast cancer. This example will help us understand how each step of the SDM model can be applied.

- **Step 1: Develop a Culture of Trust:** Jane's journey begins with her oncologist, Dr. Smith, who understands the importance of establishing trust. In their first meeting, Dr. Smith spends extra time getting to know Jane, not just as a patient but as a person with fears, hopes, and a life beyond her diagnosis. By showing genuine empathy and concern, Dr. Smith begins to build a foundation of trust. This initial interaction sets the tone for open communication, which is crucial for effective, shared decision-making.
- **Step 2: Clarity:** As they discuss Jane's condition, Dr. Smith uses clear, jargon-free language to explain the nature of breast cancer, treatment options, and potential outcomes. To aid understanding, Dr. Smith uses visual aids such as diagrams to illustrate how the cancer has affected Jane's body and what each treatment can realistically achieve. This clarity ensures Jane fully understands her medical situation, which is essential to make informed decisions about her treatment.

- **Step 3: Consideration**: With a clear understanding of her diagnosis, Jane and Dr. Smith discuss the various treatment options available, including surgery, radiation, and chemotherapy. Dr. Smith meticulously explains the benefits and risks associated with each option, allowing Jane to weigh these against her values and lifestyle. They discuss how each treatment could impact Jane's daily life, work, and family commitments, ensuring all aspects of Jane's life are considered in the decision-making process.
- **Step 4: Choice**: Finally, Jane feels prepared to make an informed decision. With Dr. Smith's support, she reflects on her priorities and chooses a treatment plan that aligns best with her desire to maintain a certain quality of life. She opts for a lumpectomy followed by radiation, which offers a balance between effective treatment and manageable side effects. This choice reflects her active participation in the decision-making process and her understanding of the potential outcomes.

This example illustrates how the 4-C Stepwise Model for Shared Decision-Making promotes a considerate, patient-focused approach to health care. By building trust, providing clarity, allowing ample time for reflection, and enabling patients to make informed decisions, health care providers can significantly improve the overall patient experience.

## The Role of Shared Decision-Making in Chronic Care

The SDM is crucial in the care of long-term illnesses. While short-term treatments may suffice for acute diseases, chronic conditions usually demand ongoing management plans that may last a patient's lifetime. Patients who participate in choosing their treatment are more inclined to follow through, resulting in improved disease management and quality of life. The concept of SDM in chronic care is not new, but it has historical origins and has been influenced by medical innovators who questioned the traditional physician-centric approach.

In the late eighteenth century, Dr. John Haygarth conducted an experiment involving wooden placebo tractors to test the efficacy of the "Perkins Tractors" metal rods, demonstrating the importance of patient engagement in medical decision-making. The findings were revolutionary: patients noted symptom improvement without medical intervention. This research illustrated the substantial impact of patient belief and participation in treatment on health results. While his main emphasis was dispelling medical misconceptions, it highlighted a key idea—patients who played an active role in their treatment choices, even though perceived options, achieved superior outcomes. His studies established an initial groundwork for contemporary comprehension of patient independence and the psychological effects of involvement in health care decisions [20].

In the early twentieth century, a significant advancement in shared decision-making was witnessed with the development of insulin for managing diabetes. Before its breakthrough in 1921 by Frederick Banting and Charles Best, type 1 diabetes often led to fatal outcomes, requiring patients to sustain themselves on starvation diets that could only prolong life for a limited time. The introduction of insulin therapy offered a pioneering yet intricate new option. Physicians were initially hesitant to widely adopt insulin due to the need for patient education, self-injection, and dietary control. This required a significant shift from passive, physician-driven care. Patients faced a choice between the new, uncertain insulin therapy and traditional restrictive diets, which prolonged life but led to severe malnutrition. Early advocates of SDM, like Dr. Elliott P. Joslin, understood the importance of patients being active participants in their diabetes care. Dr. Joslin promoted education programs to teach patients how to manage their insulin doses, monitor symptoms, and adjust treatment based on their needs [2, 24].

The use of insulin therapy was among the initial examples where the effectiveness of treatment relied heavily on patient participation, signifying an important move toward patient-focused long-term care. Diabetes management continues to be a prime example of shared decision-making, with patients and health care professionals collaboratively deciding on treatment plans considering lifestyle, individual choices, and the advancement of the disease.

A critical milestone in SDM history came with the introduction of dialysis and kidney transplantation in the 1960s. Before long-term dialysis, end-stage renal disease (ESRD) was a terminal condition. When Dr. Belding Scribner developed the arteriovenous shunt in 1960, allowing long-term dialysis, the medical community faced an unprecedented ethical dilemma—who should receive dialysis, and who should not? At the time, resources were scarce, and "Life and Death Committees" (composed of physicians, clergy, and community members) were formed to decide which patients would be selected for dialysis. However, as dialysis technology improved, the focus shifted to patient involvement in treatment choices. Patients with ESRD had to decide between dialysis and kidney transplantation, each with profound implications for quality of life.

Dr. Robert M. Arnold and Dr. Alvin Moss pioneered shared decision-making in nephrology. They highlighted the importance of patients considering the risks, benefits, and lifestyle changes related to different treatment options. Nowadays, involving patients in conversations about dialysis methods (hemodialysis vs. peritoneal dialysis) and transplant choices is fundamental to nephrology guidelines [21].

Landmark policies such as the Patient Self-Determination Act (1990) in the United States reinforced this shift by requiring health care institutions to inform patients about their rights to make medical decisions. Today, SDM is considered the gold standard in chronic disease management, ensuring patients are not passive recipients but active architects of their health care journey.

As health care continues to evolve, SDM remains essential in managing chronic diseases, empowering patients to take control of their health, and fostering a collaborative approach to medicine. By honoring the principles of SDM, medical professionals ensure medicine remains not just a science but also a shared human endeavor, where patients are treated with dignity, respect, and autonomy.

## Conclusion: The Future of Shared Decision-Making in Health Care

Shared decision-making is not just a trend; it represents a fundamental shift in how health care is delivered. As we move toward a more patient-centered health care system, the principles of shared decision-making will become increasingly important. This approach not only improves patient satisfaction and health outcomes but also enhances the overall quality of care.

The future of health care depends on our ability to connect with patients, understand their needs, and involve them in their care. By embracing shared decision-making, health care professionals can ensure they are not only providing high-quality medical care but also fostering a more compassionate and effective health care system.

Health care professionals are encouraged to integrate SDM into their daily practice to improve patient care and foster a more fulfilling and rewarding professional experience. The call to action is clear: to be medical providers who connect, influence, and empower, we must commit to shared decision-making as a core component of our practice.

**Take-Home Points**

- SDM fosters collaboration between patients and providers, enhancing satisfaction, adherence, and outcomes.
- Historical cases like Quinlan and Canterbury shaped SDM, reinforcing patient autonomy and informed consent.
- The 4-C Model (Trust, Clarity, Consideration, Choice) provides a structured approach to effective SDM.
- SDM is essential in long-term disease management, ensuring long-term adherence and personalized care.
- SDM benefits patients, providers, and health care systems by improving trust, reducing conflicts, and optimizing resource use.

## References

1. Balint M. The doctor, his patient and the illness. London: Pitman Medical Publishing; 1964.
2. Bliss M. The discovery of insulin. Chicago: The University of Chicago Press; 2013.
3. Boston Women's Health Book Collective. Our bodies, ourselves. New York: Simon and Schuster; 1973.
4. Brandt AM. Racism and research: the case of the Tuskegee syphilis study. Hast Cent Rep. 1978;8(6):21–9. https://www.ncbi.nlm.nih.gov/pubmed/721302
5. Canterbury v. Spence, No. 22099 (DC Cir. 1972). JUSTIA US Law. Retrieved February 18, 2025 from https://law.justia.com/cases/federal/appellate-courts/cadc/22099/22099.html?utm_source=chatgpt.com

6. Cassell E. The nature of suffering and the goals of medicine. New York: Oxford University Press; 1999.
7. Clark D. Between hope and acceptance: the medicalisation of dying. BMJ. 2002;324(7342):905–7. https://doi.org/10.1136/bmj.324.7342.905.
8. Coulter A. Engaging patients in health care. New York: McGraw-Hill Education; 2011.
9. Covey S. The SPEED of trust: the one thing that changes everything. New York: Free Press; 2008.
10. David Blumenthal JM. The heart of power, with a new preface: health and politics in the oval office. Berkeley: University of California Press; 2010.
11. Davis-Floyd R. Birth as an American rite of passage. Berkeley: University of California Press; 2004.
12. DeVries WC, Anderson JL, Joyce LD, Anderson FL, Hammond EH, Jarvik RK, Kolff WJ. Clinical use of the total artificial heart. N Engl J Med. 1984;310(5):273–8. https://doi.org/10.1056/NEJM198402023100501.
13. Dick-Read G. Childbirth without fear: the principles and practice of natural childbirth. London: Pinter & Martin Ltd.; 2005.
14. Eddy DM. Clinical decision making: from theory to practice. Connecting value and costs. Whom do we ask, and what do we ask them? JAMA. 1990;264(13):1737–9. https://doi.org/10.1001/jama.264.13.1737.
15. Evans DG, Barwell J, Eccles DM, Collins A, Izatt L, Jacobs C, Donaldson A, Brady AF, Cuthbert A, Harrison R, Thomas S, Howell A, FH02 Study Group, RGC teams, Miedzybrodzka Z, Murray A. The Angelina Jolie effect: how high celebrity profile can have a major impact on provision of cancer related services. Breast Cancer Res. 2014;16(5):442. https://doi.org/10.1186/s13058-014-0442-6.
16. Flexner A. The Flexner report: medical education in the United States and Canada – a report to the Carnegie Foundation for the Advancement of Teaching. Stanford: Carnegie Foundation; 1910.
17. Gawande A. Being mortal: medicine and what matters in the end. New York: Metropolitan Books; 2014.
18. Gould DB. Moving politics: emotion and ACT UP's fight against AIDS. Chicago: University of Chicago Press; 2009.
19. Groopman J. How doctors think. New York: Mariner Books; 2008.
20. Haygarth J. Of the imagination, as a cause and as a cure of disorders of the body; exemplified by fictitious tractors, and epidemical convulsions. Read to the literary and philosophical society of bath. South Carolina: Legare Street Press; 2023.
21. Hines SC, Glover JJ, Holley JL, Babrow AS, Badzek LA, Moss AH. Dialysis patients' preferences for family-based advance care planning. Ann Intern Med. 1999;130(10):825–8. https://doi.org/10.7326/0003-4819-130-10-199905180-00016.
22. Jolie A. My medical choice. The New York Times, 14 May 2013.
23. Jones JH. Bad blood: the Tuskegee syphilis experiment. New York: Free Press; 1993.
24. Joslin E. A diabetic manual for the mutual use of doctor and patient. Philadelphia: Lea & Febiger; 1941.
25. Kennedy IM. The Karen Quinlan case: problems and proposals. J Med Ethics. 1976;2(1):3–7. https://www.ncbi.nlm.nih.gov/pubmed/957371
26. Kitzinger S. The politics of birth. Books for Midwives New York: Elsevier Butterworth Heinemann; 2005.
27. Kubler-Ross E. On death and dying: what the dying have to teach doctors, nurses, clergy and their own families. New York: Scribner; 2011.
28. Kushner R. Breast cancer: a personal history and an investigative report. New York: Harcourt Brace Jovanovich; 1975.
29. Lasby C. Eisenhower's heart attack: how Ike beat heart disease and held on to the presidency. Lawrence: University Press of Kansas; 1997.
30. Lerner BH. The breast cancer wars: hope, fear, and the pursuit of a cure in twentieth-century America. Oxford: Oxford University Press; 2003.

31. Maxwell J. Developing the leader within you 2.0. Nashville: HarperCollins Leadership; 2018.
32. Millard C. Destiny of the republic: a tale of madness, medicine and the murder of a president. New York: Vintage; 2011.
33. Montori V. Why we revolt: a patient revolution for careful and kind care. Rochester: Mayo Clinic Press; 2020.
34. Montori VM, Kunneman M, Brito JP. Shared decision making and improving health care: the answer is not in. JAMA. 2017;318(7):617–8. https://doi.org/10.1001/jama.2017.10168.
35. Osler W. Aequanimitas, with other addresses to medical students, nurses and practitioners of medicine. Philadelphia: P. Blakiston's Son & Co., Inc.; 1932.
36. Peabody F. The care of the patient. JAMA. 1927. https://jamanetwork.com/journals/jama/article-abstract/245777
37. Pizer SD, Prentice JC. What are the consequences of waiting for health care in the veteran population? J Gen Intern Med. 2011;26(Suppl 2):676–82. https://doi.org/10.1007/s11606-011-1819-1.
38. Quinlan J, Quinlan J, Battelle P. Karen Ann: the Quinlans tell their story. Pennsauken: BookBaby; 2020.
39. Schweitzer A. Out of my life and thought. New York: Henry Holt and Company; 1932.
40. Shilts R. And the band played on: politics, people, and the AIDS epidemic. New York: St. Martin's Griffin; 2007.
41. Street RL Jr, Haidet P. How well do doctors know their patients? Factors affecting physician understanding of patients' health beliefs. J Gen Intern Med. 2011;26(1):21–7. https://doi.org/10.1007/s11606-010-1453-3.
42. Strub S. Body counts: a memoir of politics, sex, AIDS, and survival. New York: Scribner; 2014.
43. Szasz TS, Hollender MH. A contribution to the philosophy of medicine; the basic models of the doctor-patient relationship. AMA Arch Intern Med. 1956;97(5):585–92. https://doi.org/10.1001/archinte.1956.00250230079008.

# Part III
# Transforming Through Hope

*To offer hope is to remind someone that the future is still theirs.*

**Chapter 7: Hope**

*This final section (a single, reflective capstone) shows how all the earlier elements culminate in creating a healing presence that sustains both patient and clinician.*

# Hope

# 7

It was a calm evening in the oncology ward when Dr. Elena Martinez encountered Sarah, a 35-year-old teacher who had just received a diagnosis of an aggressive type of leukemia. Sarah was sitting quietly by the window, tightly holding a photograph of her two young daughters. Her face, pale from fatigue, reflected a sense of quiet despair. As Dr. Martinez softly introduced herself, Sarah broke the stillness with a poignant question that resonated in the sterile surroundings: "Do you think there's still hope for me?"

Dr. Martinez took a moment, reflecting on Sarah's heartfelt words. Throughout her career, she realized that while medicine has its limits, nurturing hope truly propels patients onward. "Sarah," she said gently, "hope doesn't mean turning a blind eye to our current situation. It's about faith in the potential for something brighter, even when the future feels uncertain."

Sarah took a moment before answering, her voice a bit shaky. "I'm not scared of the treatments," she said, "but I'm worried about not being there for my daughters. I promised I'd be there to see them graduate and pursue their dreams." Dr. Martinez nodded, recognizing Sarah's hope was deeply tied to her love for her family. She then shared the inspiring story of a former patient, Mia, a young mother who had bravely overcome a challenging prognosis. With her resilience, a solid support network, and relentless determination, Mia found happiness in her journey and lived long enough to welcome her first grandchild. "Hope doesn't guarantee outcomes," Dr. Martinez said, "but it opens up possibilities we may not have imagined yet."

Inspired by her conversation, Sarah embraced change. That evening, she began a journal where she penned letters to her daughters, sharing what she wanted them to know as they grew—her favorite books, the songs that brought her joy, and the lessons she hoped they would cherish. This journal became a way for Sarah to rediscover her sense of purpose.

As the weeks passed, Sarah faced many hurdles. The chemotherapy drained her energy, making some days feel like a struggle just to get out of bed. Nevertheless, she read one of her letters aloud every morning to remind herself why she was


F. Aziz, *The Healing Art of Connecting with Patients*,
https://doi.org/10.1007/978-3-032-03624-7_7

fighting. Gradually, she bonded with other patients in the ward, sharing encouraging words and lending a listening ear. Sarah's hope was contagious, creating a gentle yet strong energy that brightened the spirits of everyone nearby. One afternoon, she brought joy to the nurses by decorating the common room with drawings her daughters had sent from home. "If I can't be with them," she said with a cheerful smile, "then I can bring a little piece of them here." Her laughter echoed down the hallway, a delightful change from the heavy silence that had filled her early days in the ward.

Dr. Martinez couldn't help but admire Sarah's incredible transformation. While the path ahead remained uncertain, her change in mindset was evident. She approached her treatments with determination, asked insightful questions about her care, and took small but meaningful steps to rebuild her strength. Even her medical team observed subtle improvements in her overall health—demonstrating that hope, though hard to define, can lead to tangible results.

Months later, Sarah entered Dr. Martinez's office for her routine check-up. She appeared stronger, her eyes sparkling, and her demeanor radiated quiet confidence. "You know," she said, holding her journal, "this isn't just for my daughters anymore. It's for me, too. It serves as a reminder that life is still unfolding, even now." Sarah's journey became a powerful testament to the remarkable influence of hope—not merely as an abstract feeling but as a vital force that shapes our approach to challenges.

Let's delve into history. On a sunny September afternoon in 1848, Phineas Gage, a 25-year-old railroad foreman, was preparing for a typical day's work in Cavendish, Vermont. Gage was admired for his dedication, intelligence, and leadership qualities. His team relied on him to manage the blasting operations necessary to clear rocks for the Rutland & Burlington Railroad. During the process, Gage used a tamping iron—a lengthy, heavy metal rod—to compress gunpowder into a hole drilled in the rock. However, in an instant, a tragic accident altered the course of medical history.

During a moment of distraction, Gage made an error in the order of his actions. The tamping rod hit the rock, causing a spark that set off the gunpowder. Before anyone could react, the 13-pound iron rod, measuring 3 ft 7 in. long and 1.25 in. in diameter, shot upward like a missile, entering Gage's left cheek, passing behind his left eye, going through his brain, and exiting through the top of his skull before landing around 80 feet away. The powerful explosion knocked Gage to the ground. His co-workers, shocked by what they saw, thought he was dead. However, to their surprise, Gage survived, got up shortly after, and spoke.

Dr. John Martyn Harlow, a local physician, was surprised to find that despite his severe injuries, Gage was fully conscious and able to recount the accident. Harlow carefully examined Gage and noted the extent of his injuries, but was amazed at how alert and coherent Gage remained. Over the following weeks, Harlow closely monitored Gage's recovery, knowing infections posed a serious threat. Despite a severe abscess and delirium, Gage's strong will and careful wound care led to his remarkable recovery.

By early 1849, just a few months after the accident, Gage was physically mobile, engaging in conversations, and functioning almost normally—at least in appearance. However, those closest to him soon realized something had profoundly changed. Before the accident, Phineas Gage was known as a calm, responsible, and disciplined leader—a man his employers trusted completely. But after the injury, his personality had dramatically shifted. Harlow documented that Gage became impulsive, rude, and unable to plan effectively. He lost his social filter, often cursing and behaving in ways that were completely uncharacteristic of his former self. He could no longer hold a steady job, and his relationships suffered.

In the past, neuroscience was just starting. It was commonly thought that all parts of the brain worked the same. However, Gage's situation showed for the first time that distinct brain areas influence various aspects of personality and behavior. Recent studies indicate the iron rod harmed the left frontal lobe, which manages decision-making, impulse control, and social behavior. Gage's case was one of the first and most convincing proofs that the frontal lobe is crucial for personality and executive function.

Despite his struggles, Gage did not give up on life. Unable to return to railroad work, he embarked on a new journey—becoming one of history's most famous medical case studies. For years, he traveled around the country, giving public lectures about his survival and displaying the very iron rod that had nearly killed him. By the 1850s, he relocated to Chile, where he worked as a stagecoach driver—a job that required patience, decision-making, and responsibility. This suggests that, over time, his brain adapted, and he regained some cognitive control he had lost.

Gage eventually returned to the United States and lived with his family in California. In 1860, 12 years after his accident, he suffered a series of seizures and died at the age of 36.

Gage's case transformed our understanding of the brain. His injury and its consequences are now fundamental to modern neuroscience and psychology. His skull and the iron rod are still exhibited at the Warren Anatomical Museum at Harvard Medical School. Recent brain imaging studies have validated the nineteenth-century hypothesis that frontal lobe damage can significantly impact personality and decision-making. Phineas Gage is now honored as a remarkable survivor and a key figure in the groundbreaking medical discoveries about the human brain [24, 34].

In a different historical tale, on a crisp autumn day in 1873, Dr. Edward Livingston Trudeau was shivering in his home in New York, suffering from intense coughing spells. A skilled young physician, he had been told he had tuberculosis (TB)—a disease that was considered fatal at the time. With his elder brother already succumbing to the illness, Trudeau feared he was facing a similar fate.

Despite his medical expertise, Trudeau discovered himself descending into sadness, his physical condition deteriorating daily. The dominant medical belief at the time mainly prescribed isolation and bed rest, as most physicians thought tuberculosis was incurable. Nevertheless, a surprising development provided him with a renewed sense of determination. Acting on a friend's suggestion, Trudeau departed from the polluted atmosphere of New York City and sought refuge in the Adirondack Mountains. He hoped the clean air and peaceful surroundings would alleviate his pain.

His health improved gradually, much to his surprise. This slowed down the progression of the disease. This discovery made him realize something important: Maybe tuberculosis patients weren't hopeless. If better living conditions, fresh air, and optimism could improve his health, could they do the same for others?

Trudeau was motivated by his healing journey to embark on an ambitious mission. In 1885, he established the Adirondack Cottage Sanitarium, which was considered a groundbreaking initiative back then. He firmly believed in the power of a positive attitude, fresh air, proper nutrition, and rest to give tuberculosis patients hope. His approach was straightforward yet groundbreaking: "To cure sometimes, to relieve often, to comfort always." Trudeau's work was more than just treating tuberculosis; it was about bringing hope to those who had lost it. Patients once confined to bleak hospital rooms were now enjoying fresh mountain air, light activities, and a supportive community.

One of Trudeau's most well-known patients was a young woman named Clara, who arrived at the sanitarium in its early years. She had been given mere months to live by her previous doctors. But in the Adirondacks, she found a renewed sense of hope. Each morning, she would sit outside, bundled in blankets, watching the sunrise over the mountains. She wrote letters to her family, sharing how she felt stronger each day. Against all odds, she lived another 6 years—far longer than anyone had predicted.

Dr. Trudeau lived for 40 years following his diagnosis, during which time he saw his sanitarium become a global model for TB treatment. His contributions paved the way for contemporary pulmonary medicine, impacting the evolution of antibiotics and advanced therapies.

Trudeau's lasting legacy is a powerful reminder of the significance of hope in medicine. He recognized that doctors can provide comfort, encouragement, and belief in better days, even when a cure is unavailable. His sanitarium was a place where hope was valued as highly as medicine, a principle that still influences modern health care. Even today, Trudeau's words remind us of a fundamental truth in medicine: healing is not just about fighting disease—it's about nurturing the human spirit [22, 32].

In medicine, hope is not merely an emotion but a powerful force that can transform outcomes. It can turn despair into resilience and statistics into stories of survival. Hope is the enduring light that shines through the darkest moments, shaping patients' journeys and enhancing their quality of life. It serves as a cornerstone for healing, instilling bravery in the face of fear and resolve in the midst of hopelessness. Health care providers recognize hope as a precious asset and a vital responsibility, knowing they can nurture, inspire, and uphold it even during challenges.

## Neurobiology of Hope: Bridging Mind and Body

Hope is not just a state of mind; it's an intricate neurobiological process with tangible effects on the brain and body. The brain's reward system, mainly dopamine-dependent, is essential for experiencing hope. Dopamine—a neurotransmitter linked to motivation and pleasure—is released when we look forward to positive outcomes. This release encourages us to pursue our goals and helps us keep going, even when we face obstacles. Research using functional MRI scans indicates hopeful people show increased activity in the prefrontal cortex, the part of the brain involved in planning, decision-making, and managing emotions [5]. This brain activity implies that hope enables us to see ways to reach our goals, even during tough times.

Hope also profoundly impacts the hypothalamic-pituitary-adrenal (HPA) axis, the body's primary stress response system. Chronic stress, often a feature of serious illness, can dysregulate the HPA axis, leading to elevated levels of cortisol, a stress hormone. High cortisol levels are associated with immune suppression, inflammation, and worsened health outcomes. Hope, however, has been shown to mitigate the physiological effects of stress. By fostering optimism and reducing perceived stress, hope helps regulate the HPA axis, resulting in lower cortisol levels and a more balanced immune response [8].

On a cellular level, hope is linked to improved immune function. Studies indicate individuals with higher levels of hope have increased activity of natural killer (NK) cells, which play a critical role in combating infections and tumor cells. This enhanced immune activity highlights the mind-body connection, where positive psychological states can directly influence physical health [26].

## The Power of Hope

"Hope is life." This lovely phrase highlights the vital connection between hope and our capacity to endure and recover. It acts as a comforting yet potent force, helping individuals navigate challenging moments, providing them with the resilience to keep going and the belief that better days are ahead. Ultimately, hope is more than just a comforting dream; it is a powerful psychological tool that can significantly enhance a patient's journey through illness.

## Hope and Psychological Resilience

Hope is essential for developing psychological resilience, significantly impacting individuals who encounter challenges. People filled with hope tend to adapt more quickly to difficult situations, no matter how daunting they might appear. They usually experience lower stress, reduced anxiety, and a lower risk of depression than those lacking hope. Psychological resilience is very important for patients with complex and life-altering diagnoses. Hope can be the key to overcoming despair and successfully facing big challenges.

Viktor Frankl, a Holocaust survivor and psychiatrist, beautifully expressed this in his influential book, *Man's Search for Meaning*: "Everything can be taken from a man but one thing: the last of the human freedoms—to choose one's attitude in any given set of circumstances, to choose one's way." This perspective underscores how hope can help individuals maintain their sense of agency and dignity, even in the darkest times [14].

Charles Snyder, a prominent American psychologist who was celebrated for his contributions to positive psychology, provides a thoughtful perspective on hope. He defines it as having two essential components: agency thinking, our drive to chase our goals; and pathways thinking, the skill to create strategies to reach those goals. It's important to note that hope differs from optimism; it centers on our belief in our ability to tackle specific challenges rather than just holding a generally positive outlook. Snyder highlights hope's crucial role in our mental health, physical well-being, academic success, and overall life satisfaction, pointing out that hope is an active, goal-oriented process, not just a feeling. His theory features the Hope Scale, a tool for measurement. It suggests practical uses in education, health care, and therapy, showcasing its importance in building resilience and promoting a fulfilling life [28].

For patients and their families, fostering hope is essential. Health care providers are instrumental in encouraging this sense of positivity. Jerome Groopman, a physician and author of *The Anatomy of Hope*, says, "Hope, unlike optimism, is grounded in pure reality. It recognizes the major challenges and profound difficulties that lie ahead. Genuine hope allows no space for illusion." This realistic hope supports patients in coping and empowers them to flourish, turning their journey from simple survival into a fulfilling life [15].

Ernest Shackleton's 1914–1917 Imperial Trans-Antarctic Expedition is a remarkable tale of survival against daunting challenges. When Shackleton's ship, the Endurance, became trapped and ultimately crushed by sea ice, he and his crew found themselves stranded on the Antarctic ice. Shackleton's leadership shone through despite the harsh conditions, showcasing incredible resilience and hope. He inspired his crew to stay motivated and focused on survival, displaying an extraordinary knack for strategizing under pressure. Shackleton even undertook an audacious rescue mission, navigating 800 miles of perilous ocean to reach South Georgia Island in a small lifeboat. Remarkably, the entire crew made it through, highlighting the strength of hope and careful planning in the face of adversity. Shackleton's incredible journey is beautifully recounted in Alfred Lansing's book, *Endurance: Shackleton's Incredible Voyage*, which illustrates how hope and strong leadership can transform a dire situation into an inspiring story of survival [20].

Another uplifting story of hope and resilience during tough times is that of Louis Zamperini, whose remarkable journey is vividly portrayed in Laura Hillenbrand's biography, *Unbroken: A World War II Story of Survival, Resilience, and Redemption*.

Louis Zamperini was an Olympic track star who competed in the 1936 Berlin Olympics. Sadly, his promising athletic career was interrupted by World War II. He served as a bombardier in the United States Army Air Forces, and in 1943, his plane crashed in the Pacific Ocean during a reconnaissance mission. He survived the crash with two fellow crew members, but what followed was an extraordinary tale of survival against overwhelming odds.

Stranded on a life raft for 47 days, Zamperini and his companions faced extreme thirst and hunger, shark attacks, and the constant threat of enemy planes. Their physical limits were pushed to the brink, but Zamperini's hope and mental fortitude enabled them to endure. His leadership and steadfast spirit were vital to their survival.

Their ordeal didn't end with their rescue; upon reaching the Marshall Islands, they were captured by the Japanese Navy and spent 2 years in brutal prisoner-of-war camps. Despite enduring inhumane conditions, severe beatings, and psychological torture, Zamperini's spirit remained unbroken. His ability to cling to hope during the darkest times was essential in preserving his life and sanity.

After the war, Zamperini faced numerous challenges, including coping with post-traumatic stress disorder and feelings of anger toward his captors. However, he found solace and redemption in his faith, which reignited his hope and motivated him to become an inspiring speaker. He chose to forgive those who imprisoned him and dedicated himself to helping others navigate their struggles, demonstrating that hope can help someone through difficult times and transform deep wounds into sources of strength.

It's a powerful narrative that emphasizes the incredible impact of hope on an individual's ability to survive and thrive in light of daunting challenges [16].

## Hope as a Psychological Buffer

Hope is essential in helping patients navigate the tough feelings of fear and uncertainty that often accompany serious health diagnoses. It strikes a gentle balance between establishing realistic expectations and nurturing the possibility of positive outcomes, which is crucial to preventing a descent into hopelessness—a condition that can negatively impact both emotional and physical well-being.

Finding a good balance between enjoying the present and looking ahead with optimism is essential for our mental and emotional health, particularly when facing serious health issues. Hope acts as a potent psychological shield, aiding individuals in managing tough times by offering a sense of purpose, guidance, and resilience. For those dealing with significant health challenges, having hope can be the key to overcoming despair and approaching their recovery journey with courage and determination.

One of the most remarkable ways hope works is by serving as a protective shield against the stress and uncertainty that often come with complicated medical treatments. When patients are filled with hope, they aren't just getting by—they're getting ready to thrive. Hope empowers individuals to see beyond their present difficulties, imagining a future where their health is better and their quality of life is restored. This uplifting outlook motivates patients to take an active role in their care, transforming them from passive recipients of treatment into engaged partners in their healing journey.

I vividly remember one patient who came to me for care after undergoing a kidney transplant. Her recovery, like many others, was fraught with difficulties. There were times when her condition worsened, and the road to recovery seemed uncertain. The fear of complications and rejection was ever-present, yet her approach to these challenges was unlike most others. Despite the setbacks, she maintained an unshakable belief that she could overcome the hurdles.

This hope acted as a psychological buffer for her, protecting her from the overwhelming anxiety that could have easily derailed her progress. Instead of becoming consumed by fear, she focused on the steps she could take each day to improve her health. She adhered to her medication regimen with discipline, attended every follow-up appointment, and stayed informed about her condition. Hope was not an abstract concept for her—it was the motivation behind every decision, action, and positive change in her lifestyle.

Over time, this psychological resilience showed in tangible ways. Her kidney function stabilized, and the complications that initially seemed insurmountable became manageable. By maintaining hope, she was not only protecting her mental health but also fortifying her body's ability to heal. Hope's psychological buffer helped her face each medical challenge with a calm, focused mindset, leading to improved outcomes.

Her recovery was not just a story of physical healing but one of emotional resilience. It was a vivid illustration of how hope acts as a buffer—absorbing the stress, anxiety, and fear that often accompany serious illness and replacing them with a sense of agency and strength. By fostering hope, we enable patients to develop the psychological resilience needed to endure challenges and to see their recovery as a possibility and an achievable reality.

Through this patient's journey, I learned hope does more than inspire optimism—it creates a shield against the emotional and psychological burdens that can derail a patient's recovery. For patients facing life-altering diagnoses, hope provides the mental and emotional fortitude necessary to navigate the uncertainties of treatment. It turns what could be a passive, fearful experience into one of active participation and personal empowerment, greatly improving health outcomes and quality of life.

## Hope and Patient Engagement

Hope is more than just an emotional anchor; it actively changes how patients engage with their care, leading to better outcomes. When patients feel hopeful, they view themselves as active participants in their healing journey rather than just passive recipients of medical treatment. This shift in mindset has significant effects—hopeful patients are more likely to stick to treatment plans, attend appointments, and make positive lifestyle changes that benefit their health.

The influence of hope goes beyond individual actions; it also strengthens the relationship between patients and medical providers. Patients who are hopeful tend to build a positive and proactive connection with their medical teams, which enhances communication and leads to more personalized care. This reflects the saying: "A doctor who inspires hope inspires healing."

The patient and medical provider relationship often serves as the bedrock of hope. Patients find strength and optimism in the trust they place in their medical providers, a trust cultivated through empathy, active listening, and compassionate communication. When a medical provider creates an understanding environment, it nurtures a patient's hope and encourages greater involvement. Dr. Paul Tournier, a pioneer in psychosomatic medicine, eloquently stated: "The first duty of a doctor is to inspire hope." This principle remains fundamental to effective medical care, highlighting that healing often begins with a hopeful perspective [31].

Hope doesn't hinge on a cure or a guarantee of success. Instead, it thrives on the belief that something positive can be achieved, no matter how small. By fostering hope, health care providers empower patients to stay engaged in their care, promoting resilience and better emotional and physical outcomes.

Dr. Cicely Saunders made a significant impact on hospice care and patient engagement by emphasizing hope. Her journey in palliative care began in the 1940s when she met David Tasma, a dying Holocaust survivor, who inspired her to provide holistic care for the terminally ill. Building on her experiences as a nurse and later as a social worker, Saunders pursued medical training at St. Thomas' Hospital in London, qualifying as a physician in 1957. Her goal was clear: to improve end-of-life care by integrating pain management with compassionate support, addressing not just the physical but also the emotional, social, and spiritual needs of patients.

Dr. Saunders established St. Christopher's Hospice in London in 1967, pioneering a holistic model of care. The hospice became a hub for research and education in palliative care, shaping practices globally. Saunders introduced innovative pain control methods that enabled patients to manage pain while remaining conscious. Her groundbreaking approach viewed dying individuals as active participants in their lives until the very end.

One of Dr. Saunders' key contributions was her development of the concept of "total pain," which includes physical, emotional, social, and spiritual dimensions. She advocated for the idea that pain treatment should address all aspects of pain, recognizing that emotional and psychological support is as crucial as physical pain relief.

Her work at St. Christopher's Hospice provided a blueprint for hospice care and changed how society approaches death and dying. It fostered an environment where hope was defined not by the expectation of life prolongation but by the quality of remaining life, empowering patients to live their final days with dignity and peace [6, 9].

Henrietta Lacks, a poor African American woman from Baltimore, Maryland, became one of the most important figures in the history of medicine. However, she never lived to see the impact her life would have. Born in 1920 in the segregated South, Henrietta faced many challenges that marked her life with hardship. Still, it was her battle with cervical cancer that would lead to her profound and unintended contribution to science. Her story goes far beyond her biological contribution to medical research—it is a powerful example of patient engagement, dignity, and hope in adversity.

In 1951, Henrietta Lacks sought medical treatment at Johns Hopkins Hospital, one of the few hospitals that treated African Americans. She had been experiencing unusual symptoms, including vaginal bleeding, and after a brief examination, doctors diagnosed her with cervical cancer. During her treatment, the doctors took tissue samples from her tumor without her knowledge or consent, a practice that was common at the time. The cells from Henrietta's tumor were later cultured, creating HeLa cells, the first human cells to be successfully cultured and kept alive outside the body.

The cells quickly became invaluable to researchers, contributing to cancer research breakthroughs, the polio vaccine's development, and advancements in gene mapping. However, Henrietta Lacks never knew the role her cells would play in revolutionizing medical science. She was never informed about the use of her cells, and her family was left unaware for many years about the importance of what had been taken from her.

Despite this lack of informed consent, Henrietta's engagement with her care during her brief life was one of incredible strength. She underwent radiation treatment, which caused significant pain and discomfort, but she remained focused on her family and her life. It was reported that, even in her last days, she held on to the hope that she would survive her illness and be able to live longer for the sake of her children. However, in August 1951, Henrietta died from complications of the cancer, but her cells lived on, growing exponentially in labs around the world.

Though Henrietta's story remained largely unknown for decades, her legacy was recognized after her death, largely thanks to the investigative work of Rebecca Skloot. Skloot's book not only revealed the scientific achievements that came from the use of Henrietta's cells but also focused on the ethical issues surrounding her treatment, including the exploitation of African Americans in medical research and the violation of her fundamental rights as a patient. Skloot's investigation also highlighted the struggles of Henrietta's family, who were never compensated for using her cells and were unaware of her contribution to modern science until years later.

Her family's journey of understanding the significance of Henrietta's contribution also highlights the evolving relationship between patients and health care providers. The discovery that Henrietta's cells had been taken without her consent sparked a national conversation about the rights of patients, especially those from marginalized communities. Her story became a catalyst for policy changes in the way medical research is conducted today. In particular, the case brought attention to the need for informed consent in medical procedures, establishing legal and ethical frameworks for handling patient tissue and information.

The legacy of Henrietta Lacks is one of both scientific progress and the struggle for patient rights. Her story reminds us that while hope can empower patients to engage with their care, it must be built on trust, transparency, and respect for patient autonomy. She was not only a passive subject of medical research but a symbol of the untapped potential of every patient's story. Her life and the discovery of HeLa cells are powerful testimonies to the idea that patients, even under challenging circumstances, possess the resilience and hope necessary to endure and change the world in ways they may never see.

As a society, the story of Henrietta Lacks teaches us that fostering patient engagement is about much more than just compliance with medical advice. It's about providing patients with hope, dignity, and agency in their health care journey. Her experience, both tragic and triumphant, continues to inspire health care providers to view patients as active participants in their care and to ensure their contributions—whether through research or resilience—are acknowledged and respected [27].

## The Relentless Nature of Hope

Emily Dickinson beautifully captured the essence of hope when she said it is "the thing with feathers that perches in the soul—and sings the tune without the words—and never stops at all." This lovely metaphor highlights the unwavering and persistent nature of hope. It is a quiet, reliable force that remains strong, even when faced with tough challenges, especially in medical environments. For patients enduring long or difficult treatments, hope acts as a stabilizing anchor, helping them navigate through uncertainty and discomfort [11].

Hope offers the emotional strength necessary to tackle challenging journeys. It becomes a gentle, encouraging voice, urging patients to hang on and push through for just one more day as the possibility of a brighter future always lingers. Hope inspires this personal growth, helping patients adapt and discover meaning even in their most challenging times.

In the clinical realm, the power of hope is crucial for healing. Research indicates hope is closely linked to enhanced psychological well-being and better adherence to treatment. Patients who maintain hope are more inclined to follow medical advice, keep a positive attitude, and stay motivated throughout their treatment journey [29].

To further illustrate the relentless nature of hope, particularly in challenging medical contexts, the historical story of Norman Cousins is highly inspirational. Cousins was an editor and a long-time advocate for world peace and patient rights, whose story is detailed in his book, *Anatomy of an Illness as Perceived by the Patient.*

In 1964, Norman Cousins faced a challenging diagnosis of ankylosing spondylitis, a serious form of arthritis. Despite the grim outlook, he remained hopeful and devised a unique recovery plan. Cousins opted for unconventional methods, such as high doses of Vitamin C and laughter therapy, by watching Candid Camera episodes and Marx Brothers films in a hotel instead of the hospital.

Cousins believed negative emotions could worsen illness, while positive emotions could help fight it. His self-created treatment led to a notable decrease in pain and a slow recovery, giving him insights into how emotions impact the body's biochemistry and the potential of a positive mindset in influencing disease recovery. His remarkable recovery was not just a medical anomaly but a true testament to the incredible power of hope and the mind-body connection. Despite doctors predicting his imminent demise, Cousins returned to work at the Saturday Review magazine and lived for another 26 years. During this time, he dedicated himself to advocating for a more holistic approach to patient care, underscoring the importance of the human side of medicine.

Norman Cousins' experience demonstrates the significant impact of hope in dealing with illness. It highlights the importance of maintaining a positive outlook on health, showing how it can influence the body's response to disease and treatment. His story proves hope can motivate patients to seek healing, even while facing daunting health obstacles [10].

Lance Armstrong, the celebrated American cyclist, is another powerful example of the relentless nature of hope and its transformative impact on health outcomes. Armstrong's story is not just about his extraordinary achievements in cycling but also about his battle with cancer and how hope, combined with perseverance, can overcome even the most severe challenges.

In 1996, Armstrong was diagnosed with advanced testicular cancer that had spread to his brain and lungs. The prognosis was grim. Doctors gave him a mere 40% chance of survival. Yet, throughout his treatment, Armstrong remained resolute in his hope for recovery. He decided he would not succumb to despair and, instead, he would fight with every ounce of his being.

Armstrong showed unwavering determination during his treatment, including surgery and chemotherapy. His ability to maintain a positive and forward-looking mindset set him apart. He wrote about how, during his chemotherapy sessions, he would visualize himself crossing the finish line at the Tour de France, the pinnacle of cycling achievement. This visualization of a hopeful future helped him endure the pain and exhaustion of treatment, reinforcing the power of hope as a motivator.

Armstrong's resilience during treatment was extraordinary. Despite the debilitating effects of chemotherapy, he pushed forward with the belief he would recover and return to cycling. His hope was not just a passive wish—it was an active driving force that helped him maintain mental clarity and emotional strength during the most physically and mentally taxing moments of his life.

In 1999, just 3 years after his diagnosis, Armstrong made a stunning comeback by winning the Tour de France for the first time. His victory was a triumph of athleticism and a testament to the incredible power of hope in overcoming illness. Armstrong went on to win the prestigious race seven times, a record that has cemented his place in cycling history. His story of survival and success captivated millions around the world and became a symbol of hope for cancer patients everywhere.

Armstrong also founded the Lance Armstrong Foundation, LIVESTRONG, to support survivors and promote cancer awareness. His foundation has helped millions worldwide and shows how one individual's hope and determination can inspire others to take control of their health and fight for a brighter future.

While Armstrong's story is often remembered for his athletic success, it is also a compelling reminder of the relentless nature of hope. For patients battling life-threatening conditions, hope is not just an emotional reaction but a necessary tool in their fight for survival. Armstrong's journey shows that hope can be a powerful force that propels patients forward, even when the odds seem insurmountable. His recovery and subsequent advocacy work have inspired countless individuals, highlighting the profound connection between mental resilience, emotional strength, and physical recovery [19].

## Hope and the Placebo Effect

The incredible power of hope shines through in the placebo effect, where a patient's belief in a treatment's effectiveness—even when it contains no real active ingredients—can lead to genuine improvements in their health. This fascinating relationship between belief and biology shows how much hope can impact physical well-being.

This "biology of hope" highlights the close connection between our minds and bodies. When patients feel hopeful, their mental state can positively affect their physical health, often leading to better outcomes than anticipated. Research has demonstrated that the placebo effect can cause notable changes, such as pain relief, mood enhancement, and even normalizing biological markers like blood pressure and heart rate [4]. This shows hope is more than just a mental concept; it has real physical effects.

For instance, in clinical trials, patients given a placebo frequently report significant symptom relief, not due to the treatment itself but because they believe they are being cared for and that improvement is within reach. This is a powerful reminder that hope is more than just wishful thinking—it triggers real biological changes. The release of endorphins, dopamine, and other neurotransmitters in response to hope and positive expectations initiates a healing process in the body [5].

This deep connection between hope and the body's healing abilities encourages medical providers to think about how their words and actions can nurture hope in their patients. Simple gestures, like reassuring or showing empathy, can enhance the placebo effect and strengthen the therapeutic relationship.

Dr. Henry Beecher, an anesthesiologist and a pioneer in pain management research, first became interested in the placebo effect during World War II while serving as a medic. He noticed injured soldiers frequently experienced less pain than anticipated, given the extent of their wounds. This led Beecher to explore the connection between expectation, belief, and pain sensitivity in soldiers.

One significant moment occurred when Beecher ran out of morphine after a battle and had to conduct surgeries and medical procedures using saline injections instead. Surprisingly, many soldiers noted considerable pain relief from these saline injections, thinking they had been given morphine. This incident prompted Beecher to suggest that the soldiers' expectations influenced their pain experience, a concept he later named the "placebo effect."

After the war, Beecher kept investigating this phenomenon. In 1955, he released a groundbreaking paper titled "The Powerful Placebo." In this paper, Beecher revealed that in 15 different clinical trials, an average of 35% of patients found relief from different ailments after receiving a placebo treatment. This study transformed how clinical trials were conducted, introducing control groups and placebo treatments as standard procedures and underscoring the biological underpinnings of hope and belief [4].

Beecher's research showed that having hope can significantly impact physical health, leading to real improvements in health even without medical treatment. This finding is important for health care, highlighting how patient beliefs and expectations play a key role in healing. It suggests that promoting hope and positivity can significantly improve treatment results.

In recent years, researchers have continued to explore the placebo effect, discovering how the power of belief and hope can lead to significant improvements in health. One particularly fascinating study conducted by researchers at Harvard Medical School in 2010 delved into the potential of an "open-label placebo"—a placebo treatment in which patients are fully aware they are receiving a placebo. The study challenged the conventional understanding that a placebo only works when the patient believes they are receiving an effective treatment, revealing the profound effects of hope and expectation on the body's healing process.

The research, led by Dr. Ted Kaptchuk, a professor of medicine at Harvard, aimed to explore whether patients explicitly told they were taking a placebo could still experience the therapeutic benefits commonly associated with placebo treatments. The study involved 80 patients suffering from irritable bowel syndrome (IBS), a condition that often has no clear treatment. Half of the patients were given a placebo pill, while the other half received no treatment. All participants were informed that the pill was a placebo, yet the patients who received it reported significant improvements in their symptoms, including reduced pain and discomfort.

This open-label placebo study demonstrated that knowing they received a placebo did not negate the benefits. The hope and belief in improvement were still enough to trigger genuine biological changes in the body. The patients' physical symptoms improved not because of the pills themselves but because of their expectations and the belief that the treatment would help them. This finding challenges the traditional notion that the placebo effect is solely a result of deceiving patients. Instead, it suggests the simple act of receiving care and expecting improvement can trigger physiological changes in the body, underlining the incredible power of hope.

The research on open-label placebos further emphasizes how hope and belief are integral components of healing, showcasing how belief can trigger biochemical responses like the release of endorphins, dopamine, and other neurotransmitters that promote pain relief and overall wellness. This development in placebo research reaffirms the mind-body connection and encourages health care professionals to consider the psychological and emotional dimensions of treatment alongside the physical ones [18].

## The Therapeutic Power of Hope

For those navigating the challenges of a long-term illness, hope acts as an essential lifeline. It offers the mental and emotional strength required to face the unpredictable ups and downs of their condition. Hope inspires patients to stay dedicated to living life to the fullest, even when physical and emotional hurdles arise. It turns feelings of despair into a strong sense of determination and nurtures resilience in the most challenging times.

Hope is truly contagious. When medical providers share and radiate hope during their interactions with patients, it can create a positive ripple effect that reaches the patient and their family and wider support network. This shared sense of hope cultivates a warm atmosphere where patients feel supported, understood, and inspired to keep going. By expressing hope through their words and actions, medical providers strengthen the therapeutic bond and motivate patients to be involved in their care and stay optimistic.

Paul Kalanithi's journey is an extraordinary and poignant reminder of the power of hope, resilience, and purpose, even when facing the relentless progression of terminal illness. Kalanithi, a talented neurosurgeon and aspiring writer, was diagnosed with stage IV lung cancer at the age of 36. At the time, he was nearing the completion of his training in neurosurgery and had a promising future ahead of him. Instead of the anticipated joy of beginning his career, he found himself thrust into the world he had devoted his life to understanding—suffering, illness, and death.

His diagnosis was a devastating blow. In a profession dedicated to saving lives and curing diseases, Kalanithi, who had spent years studying the intricacies of the human brain, now had to confront his mortality. Lung cancer, particularly in its late stages, was a death sentence. The prospect of living only a few more years or months hung heavily over him.

However, instead of succumbing to despair, Kalanithi faced his diagnosis with courage, deep reflection, and an unwavering belief in the possibility of finding meaning and hope—even in the face of the inevitable. In the months following his diagnosis, Kalanithi experienced the full range of emotions: grief, fear, anger, and acceptance. Yet, through it all, he kept returning to one fundamental question: What is the meaning of life, especially when death is near? His work as a neurosurgeon had allowed him to witness the fragility of life in ways few people could comprehend. But now, as a patient, he was forced to confront his mortality and the choices he would have to make in the time he had left.

During his treatment, Kalanithi found profound solace in his work and the relationships he maintained with his patients. His understanding of death as a physician and a patient gave him a unique perspective on the human experience. As he wrote in his memoir, *When Breath Becomes Air*, "Even when we know that we can't control the outcome, we can control our response." This belief became the cornerstone of his resilience. Despite his worsening condition, Kalanithi chose to continue living with purpose, focusing on what he could contribute to the world, even in his limited time.

One of the most profound aspects of Kalanithi's story is his continued practicing medicine despite his diagnosis. He remained committed to caring for his patients, providing the same compassion and expertise he had always offered. Even as his health deteriorated, he found strength in the connection between doctor and patient. He saw the power of healing not just in medical treatments but in the human connection, in the ability to comfort, listen, and be present with others in their time of need.

As the disease progressed, Kalanithi's focus shifted more and more toward his family, particularly his wife, Lucy, and their young daughter, whom they had recently welcomed into the world. In his final months, he reflected deeply on the significance of family, love, and legacy. His desire to be a good father, husband, and doctor drove his ability to keep fighting. Despite his pain and the inevitable progression of his illness, he remained determined to be there for his family, to live as fully as possible, and to leave behind a legacy of love, care, and meaning.

Kalanithi's memoir was written during the final stages of his life, and its publication after his death brought his story to a broader audience. Through his writing, Kalanithi explored the intersection of science, philosophy, and the human experience, offering a powerful meditation on what it means to live a meaningful life, especially when faced with death. His reflections on his illness and his work as a physician offer profound insights into the role of hope in chronic disease. Even as his body weakened, Kalanithi's mind remained sharp and engaged, focused on creating meaning from his remaining time [17].

The therapeutic power of hope is immense. It connects despair with resilience, motivating patients and their communities to move forward, even when facing a long-term illness. By nurturing hope, health care providers play a vital role in helping their patients reclaim control over their lives, promoting survival and a significant and thriving existence.

## The Physician's Role in Cultivating Hope

The role of a medical provider goes beyond simply using medical knowledge; it's about supporting patients during some of their most challenging times. In this light, hope plays a vital role in providing adequate care. Medical providers are not only healers of the body but also guardians of hope, a quality that can significantly impact a patient's emotional and physical experience while dealing with illness.

### The Dual Imperative: Honesty and Hope

One of the most challenging jobs for a medical provider is finding the right balance between sharing honest information and nurturing hope. This balance is key to the relationship between patients and their medical providers. In a clinical setting, sharing difficult news—about a diagnosis, prognosis, or treatment limitations—is an unavoidable and often challenging part of the role. However, how this news is conveyed can significantly influence a patient's reaction, resilience, and outlook.

Dr. Bernard Lown, a Nobel laureate and esteemed cardiologist, pointed out, "The most essential quality for the clinician is not technical skill, but compassion" [23]. This compassion is vital when walking the fine line between truth and hope. Patients deserve to have clear and transparent information about their condition, as this is crucial for making informed decisions and planning realistically. At the same time, it's important that this reality doesn't extinguish hope but rather exists alongside it. Hope helps patients find strength and purpose, even when facing tough challenges, enhancing their ability to cope and engage in care.

Hope doesn't mean giving false reassurance or downplaying the seriousness of a situation. Instead, it's about presenting the truth in a way that brings attention to potential opportunities, strengths, and paths forward. For instance, when discussing a difficult prognosis, medical providers might highlight available treatment options, advancements in research, or clinical trials that could open new doors for care. Beyond medical possibilities, hope can also stem from recognizing the patient's personal resilience, support system, or small but significant achievements along the way.

This approach isn't just about emotions; it's practical, too, as hope has been shown to positively affect health outcomes. In Charles Snyder's words, "a mindset that allows us to perceive that we can control our future" [29]. By nurturing this mindset, medical providers can empower patients to feel a sense of hope, which is essential for their mental and emotional health.

A powerful modern-day illustration of practicing hope in medicine unfolded during the height of the COVID-19 pandemic—a time marked by uncertainty, isolation, and overwhelming loss. On Thanksgiving Day in November 2020, Dr. Joseph Varon, Chief of Critical Care at United Memorial Medical Center in Houston, was making his usual rounds in the COVID-19 intensive care unit. Like every other day in the ICU, the air was thick with anxiety, and the atmosphere was somber. But something stopped him in his tracks: an elderly patient, visibly distressed, sitting on the edge of his hospital bed, sobbing.

This patient, separated from his family and community by necessary but isolating infection protocols, had reached an emotional breaking point. The relentless solitude, combined with the gravity of his illness, had left him feeling completely alone. He told Dr. Varon through tears, "I want to be with my wife." Moved by the sheer human pain in front of him, Dr. Varon did something deeply instinctive and compassionate—he stepped forward and embraced the patient. Despite being fully suited in layers of PPE, he reached out not just as a physician but as a fellow human being.

The moment was captured in a photo by journalist Go Nakamura—a physician hugging a crying patient in full pandemic gear—and the image went viral. It became a global symbol of what it truly means to care. Dr. Varon would later reflect, "This man was crying, and I just didn't know what to say. So I gave him a hug" [12].

What Dr. Varon demonstrated so profoundly in that moment was the essential tension every clinician must navigate: the balance between reality and hope. He couldn't change the medical facts. The patient was seriously ill, and the prognosis was uncertain. But he *could* offer presence, empathy, and an emotional anchor in a time of despair. He didn't provide false reassurance. He didn't deny the reality of the illness. Instead, he stood with the patient in that reality and brought a flicker of hope into it—not through words, but through connection.

In Dr. Varon's hug, the world saw not just an act of kindness but a philosophy of care. It was a moment that affirmed how medicine, at its core, is not just about curing disease but about caring for people. And in that embrace, we are reminded that the delicate balance between reality and hope is not a compromise but a commitment to honor the truth while nurturing the human spirit.

## Empathic Communication: The Bridge to Hope

Empathic communication is essential in creating a connection that balances honesty with hope. It goes beyond merely sharing facts; it requires a genuine understanding of the patient's feelings, recognizing their fears, and offering compassionate support that is both realistic and uplifting. When empathy is present, trust flourishes, forming the foundation for hope in health care settings. Patients who feel truly heard are much more likely to muster the emotional resilience needed to confront their challenges and stay engaged in their treatment.

Fogarty et al. discovered that patients who experienced empathy from their health care providers not only reported improved emotional well-being but also felt more hopeful and satisfied with their care [13]. Active listening is crucial in establishing this bond. Although it may seem straightforward, active listening demands genuine focus, patience, and presence—qualities that can be tough to maintain in a busy medical environment. However, dedicating time to listen and validate a patient's feelings can significantly shift their perspective.

## The Therapeutic Alliance: Building a Foundation of Trust

The relationship between a doctor and a patient is one of health care's most powerful yet often overlooked aspects. This connection, built on trust, respect, and a shared dedication to the patient's health, is fundamental to effective care. A solid therapeutic alliance goes beyond just facilitating communication; it becomes a vital source of hope and resilience for the patient.

At the core of this relationship is trust. Patients need to believe their medical provider is not only skilled but also genuinely cares about their well-being. This trust is nurtured through expertise, empathetic communication, and authentic concern. Technical ability alone isn't enough—patients must feel understood and acknowledged in their worries, fears, and hopes. As Francis Peabody wisely noted in his famous 1927 speech, "The secret of the care of the patient is in caring for the patient" [25]. This highlights the important truth that effective care addresses not just physical health but also the emotional and psychological aspects of a patient's experience.

During the 2014–2016 Ebola outbreak in West Africa, clinicians faced not only one of the most dangerous viruses known to humankind but also a deep crisis of trust. In countries like Sierra Leone, Liberia, and Guinea, many citizens were skeptical of government institutions and foreign health workers. Rumors spread rapidly: that Ebola was a hoax, hospitals were killing people, those in hazmat suits were harvesting organs. Without clear, compassionate communication, fear became the dominant narrative—and hope became elusive.

As a result, many infected individuals chose to stay home rather than seek treatment, and entire communities hid symptomatic loved ones. Medical workers weren't welcomed—they were feared. This mistrust, fueled by historical trauma and poor communication, severely hampered efforts to contain the disease. Patients refused testing, rejected isolation, and avoided life-saving care. Despite the best intentions of health care teams, they could not make progress because their offers of help were not believed.

Enter Dr. Javid Abdelmoneim, a British-Sudanese physician working with Médecins Sans Frontières (Doctors Without Borders). When he arrived in Sierra Leone, he quickly understood that delivering medical treatment wasn't enough—he and his team had to first earn the right to care, which required building trust, one patient at a time.

Working in sweltering temperatures inside stifling PPE, unable to offer the kind of human touch that usually communicates care, Abdelmoneim and his team found creative ways to reconnect. They began using whiteboards to write patients' names on the walls of their treatment tents—small acts that gave back identity and dignity. They updated families daily, often through community liaisons, making sure that even the sickest patients were never invisible. The team also explained procedures slowly and clearly, often with the help of trusted local interpreters, countering misinformation with consistency and patience.

One of the most striking shifts came when a patient who had initially refused care began to trust the team after repeated kind interactions. "He started talking to us, asking questions, showing signs that he wanted to live," Dr. Abdelmoneim recalled. "And from that point on, he fought. And he survived."

It wasn't a miracle drug or a new protocol that saved him—it was hope born from trust. In this fragile, high-stakes environment, trust became the lifeline that connected patients to their care, to their families, and to their will to survive.

This story reminds us that trust is not just about believing in science—it's about believing in the person delivering it. For patients to hold onto hope, they need to know they are seen, heard, and safe. Without trust, care cannot begin. It makes healing possible—even in the darkest moments [1].

## Hope in Chronic Medical Conditions

Chronic illness has the power to slowly diminish a patient's sense of self, security, and agency. Despite the challenges of medical tests, treatments, uncertainty, and moments of solitude, hope frequently emerges as a potent force in a patient's journey. This hope is not blind positivity or false comfort; rather, it is the belief that life, even in sickness, can still offer purpose, significance, and happiness. In medical practice, we witness how hope enables patients to persevere—whether through chemotherapy, dialysis, immunosuppressants, or pain management routines. It serves as their guiding light, shaping their perspective and often influencing their outcomes. The narratives shared—covering cancer, chronic kidney disease, and autoimmune conditions—underscore that hope is not a luxury but a crucial component of recovery, a form of silent therapy, and one of the most valuable gifts a health care provider can help nurture.

## Hope as a Catalyst in Cancer Care

In cancer patients, hope is more than just passing emotional support; it is often the foundation for sticking to treatment, bouncing back from challenges, and maintaining a good quality of life. Studies reveal that hope can enhance mental well-being, boost the immune system, and encourage active participation in treatment, even in the face of tough side effects or unclear outcomes. However, the real impact of hope is best seen through individual experiences.

In 2013, Roselyn Singleton, a Navy veteran from North Carolina, was diagnosed with brain cancer. After undergoing a craniotomy to remove a tumor, she entered remission. But her life was turned upside down again in 2019 when the cancer returned—this time more aggressively.

Despite the diagnosis, Roselyn chose to face each day with strength and intentional joy. Her husband, Ray Singleton, began recording candid, heartfelt videos of their life together—often featuring him singing while she sat in the background, smiling or dancing. These moments, shared online during the early days of the COVID-19 pandemic, captured hearts worldwide. Roselyn became known not just as a cancer patient but as a symbol of courage, grace, and hope.

Her hope wasn't rooted in denial of her diagnosis. It was grounded in the everyday goals she set: celebrating anniversaries, supporting other cancer patients, speaking publicly, and finding meaning in her life despite her illness. In 2020, the couple appeared on *The Ellen DeGeneres Show*, where Ellen praised Roselyn's outlook and helped raise awareness for brain cancer support.

Roselyn died in 2022, but not before fulfilling many of her personal goals and touching the lives of thousands. In a 2021 interview, she said: "I may have cancer, but cancer does not have me. Hope means I still get to choose how I live."

Her journey illustrates the profound connection between trust, love, and purposeful hope—and how these forces can anchor a patient through even the most uncertain outcomes [21].

In early 2020, just as the COVID-19 pandemic was reshaping health care worldwide, a 22-year-old woman was diagnosed with Hodgkin's lymphoma. Her treatment was scheduled at Memorial Sloan Kettering Cancer Center (MSK), one of the nation's premier oncology institutions. However, as lockdowns escalated, hospitals implemented strict visitor restrictions, and supply chains for chemotherapy agents became strained. Many young adult patients faced delays and emotional disconnection when support was critical.

Rather than give in to despair, she turned to writing as a coping mechanism. Supported by MSK's Adolescent and Young Adult (AYA) Program, she began journaling daily. Eventually, she started writing poems about her experience—about her hair loss, her fear, and the isolation of fighting cancer in a pandemic. Her oncologist, impressed by her creative expression and emotional resilience, encouraged her to submit her work to ASCO Voices. On this platform, patients and clinicians share potent narratives from the frontlines of cancer care.

She also created short-term goals to keep herself motivated: finish her poetry collection, walk every day when not too fatigued, and attend her college graduation—virtually if necessary. These simple but meaningful aspirations provided a roadmap for emotional survival and gave her something to fight for on days when her body was weak, but her spirit still flickered with hope.

In 2021, she entered remission. She completed her treatment, published her poetry online, and gave a virtual talk during AYA Cancer Awareness Week. In her closing words, she shared: “Hope, to me, wasn’t about thinking everything would be okay. It was about believing there was still something worth holding on to, even in the hardest moments.” Her story affirms what cancer clinicians have long observed: patients with hope do more than survive—they engage, connect, and sometimes inspire others to live more fully [30].

Stories like Roselyn’s show hope is not about denying reality but about standing strong against despair. It is based on love, purpose, and connection. For cancer patients, nurturing hope is not just a nice gesture—it is crucial for their well-being.

## Hope in the Journey of Chronic Kidney Disease

Dealing with chronic kidney disease (CKD) is not just a physical struggle, but it also brings emotional and existential challenges. Patients relying on dialysis or waiting for a transplant find their daily routines revolving around machines, medical tests, and simply staying alive. The emotional toll of fatigue, loneliness, lifestyle changes, and facing mortality can feel like a heavy burden. However, hope frequently emerges as a powerful force that enables patients to regain control, redefine themselves, and reconnect with life.

In 2019, Robert Chelsea made medical history as the first African American and the oldest person (age 68) to receive a full face transplant. His path to that groundbreaking moment was shaped not just by surgery but by a long, silent battle with chronic illness, including end-stage renal disease.

In 2013, Robert was critically injured in a car crash when a drunk driver struck his vehicle. He suffered burns over more than 60% of his body, including severe disfigurement to his face. What followed were years of pain, multiple surgeries, and unforeseen complications—including kidney failure, which forced him onto dialysis while waiting for a face transplant. Dialysis became a defining part of his routine and, at times, a limiting factor in his eligibility for reconstructive procedures.

Yet Robert remained grounded in a sense of purpose. In interviews, he often described his faith, his love for his daughter, and the hope of reentering the world without shame as driving forces in his recovery. “I want to be present for my daughter’s life,” he said. “And if my story can help others, it’s worth sharing.”

He was fiercely adherent to his dialysis schedule and post-operative protocols, even when they were exhausting. That discipline and belief eventually made it possible for him to receive both a kidney transplant and a face transplant, making his recovery one of the most inspiring and medically complex in recent history.

Robert’s story is not only about medical innovation—it is about how hope, rooted in identity, family, and faith, can sustain a person through the darkest corridors of illness. His resilience redefines what it means to live with CKD—not simply to survive but to transform [7].

The importance of hope in the CKD journey is profoundly illustrated in the children's book *Maria Never Gives Up: Are You Brave Like Me?* by Mary Baliker. Based on real-life experiences, the story follows Maria, a vibrant young girl suddenly diagnosed with kidney disease. Her world changes overnight. She is now a patient—required to navigate a maze of hospital visits, unfamiliar procedures, and the physical discomfort of treatments she can barely pronounce.

In the beginning, Maria is frightened. Her energy is low. She feels different from her classmates. Questions flood her mind—*Why me? Will I always feel like this? Will I be okay?* These are not just questions children ask; they echo what many adult patients feel, often in silence. But Maria's story doesn't end in fear. With the help of her loving parents, a wise and comforting teddy bear, and a team of compassionate clinicians, she begins to confront her illness not as an end, but as a challenge she can face with bravery.

What changes for Maria is not her disease, but her perspective. She starts setting small goals: getting through a blood draw without tears, attending school even when tired, and learning to explain her condition to others. As her confidence grows, so does her sense of control. She begins to feel proud of her resilience and starts encouraging other children in the hospital. She becomes, in essence, a beacon of hope—not only for herself but for others around her.

In one pivotal scene, Maria looks into the mirror and says, "I may be sick, but I am not weak. I am strong. I am brave. I am me." This simple affirmation captures a deeper psychological truth: Hope takes root when patients reclaim their narrative and see themselves beyond the diagnosis.

Even in the face of an incurable condition, hope becomes a lifeline—not through denial of the disease, but through the determination to live fully with it. Maria teaches us all—regardless of age—that illness can be a part of your story, but it doesn't have to define your story. And as she bravely declares in her final pages: "No matter how hard it gets, I will never give up. And maybe, just maybe, you won't either" [3].

These stories—one shaped by groundbreaking surgery, the other by quiet resilience in a virtual room—remind us that hope is not abstract. It is found in faith, family, shared experience, and small but meaningful goals. For patients with CKD, hope is not about denying the difficulties of treatment. Rather, it is the belief that life can still hold purpose, joy, and connection. And that belief, nurtured by clinicians, families, and communities, can transform compliance into commitment and survival into living.

## Autoimmune Disorders: Hope as a Force of Stability and Meaning

Living with autoimmune conditions such as lupus, rheumatoid arthritis, and multiple sclerosis can make daily life unpredictable. Dealing with these lifelong illnesses goes beyond medication; it demands a hopeful outlook. Embracing hope is a powerful mental strategy.

In 2015, at the height of her musical and acting career, Selena Gomez shocked fans by revealing she had been quietly battling systemic lupus erythematosus. At first, she kept her diagnosis private, undergoing chemotherapy and treatment while still touring. But behind the scenes, her health was deteriorating—lupus was attacking her kidneys, and by 2017, her doctors told her she needed a kidney transplant.

What happened next changed not only her health but her entire relationship with her illness. Her close friend, actress Francia Raisa, offered to donate her kidney. The transplant was a success, but the emotional aftermath—fear, pain, anxiety—was still overwhelming. Rather than retreat, Selena stepped forward, using her global platform to raise awareness about lupus, mental health, and the emotional toll of living with invisible illness.

In her 2022 documentary *My Mind & Me*, Selena not only speaks openly about moments of hopelessness and frustration but also about the power of purpose. She founded the Rare Impact Fund to support mental health services and has partnered with the Lupus Research Alliance to advocate for better treatments. "Hope isn't always easy," she says in the film. "But every time I meet someone who says my story helped them feel less alone, I remember why I keep going."

Selena's story illustrates how hope is sustained by internal strength, the meaning-making community, and the decision to live transparently. She turned a deeply personal struggle into a public mission, reminding millions that life can still be purposeful and joyful even in the face of chronic illness [2, 33].

In 2020, as the COVID-19 pandemic gripped the world, 29-year-old Elena, a freelance graphic designer in the UK, faced a dual crisis: worsening rheumatoid arthritis symptoms and sudden disruption of her routine care. Her infusions were delayed, rheumatology clinic visits were moved online, and she was advised to shield due to her immunosuppressed state. Alone in her apartment and unsure of what the next day might bring, Elena described those early pandemic months as some of the most terrifying of her life.

Her physical pain intensified. Simple tasks like opening a jar or typing for long hours became painful. But the real battle was emotional—grief over lost independence, anxiety over infections, and a creeping hopelessness.

That's when she discovered a virtual peer support group through the UK charity Versus Arthritis. At first, she was hesitant to join. But in those weekly sessions, filled with people who *understood* her pain without explanation, she felt seen. One member recommended journaling. Another shared their routine for managing flares. Eventually, Elena began writing and sharing her own experiences online.

She launched a modest Instagram account—@ChronicallyElena—where she shared creative graphics about invisible illness, mobility, and mental health. Her account quickly gained traction. "People told me they didn't feel so alone anymore," she said in a 2021 interview with Versus Arthritis. "But the truth is—they were giving *me* hope."

Over time, her mood lifted. Her self-care habits improved. She resumed regular physiotherapy and found renewed energy in art, advocacy, and community. "I still have RA," Elena says, "but I no longer feel like it has me."

Her journey is a testament to the idea that hope isn't denying difficulty—it's the decision to keep engaging with life, even when it hurts.

Both Selena and Elena show us that hope doesn't emerge passively—it is cultivated. It arises when patients are supported, empowered, and invited to create meaning beyond their illness. Whether through advocacy, peer support, or personal storytelling, hope gives patients with autoimmune disorders the emotional grounding to persist through unpredictability—and even transform their pain into purpose.

## Conclusion

Hope is not a cure but often the beginning of healing. It is the quiet force that allows patients to face uncertainty with courage, transforming despair into resilience and fear into purpose. From cancer wards to dialysis centers, from ancient sanitariums to modern ICUs, the stories shared in this chapter reveal hope is not passive—it is active, cultivated through compassion, trust, and connection. For medical providers, offering hope is not about guaranteeing outcomes; it is about walking beside patients, honoring their journey, and reminding them that even in the darkest moments, something meaningful still lies ahead.

**Take-Home Points**

- Hope is a critical psychological anchor that improves treatment adherence and emotional resilience.
- Empathic communication fosters trust, essential for sustaining hope in clinical care.
- Hope is not false reassurance—it is the honest belief in possibility amid uncertainty.
- Patient stories reveal that hope often emerges through connection, purpose, and personal goals.
- Medical providers can nurture hope by being present, listening deeply, and honoring the whole person—not just the disease.

## References

1. Abdelmoneim J. Ebola: the British doctor on the front line. 2014. Retrieved March 31, 2025, from https://www.bbc.com/news/uk-30054775
2. Bailey A. Selena Gomez on the moment she realized 'all of these years of confusion and being in love' were worth It. 2022. https://www.elle.com/culture/celebrities/a34703935/selena-gomez-newsette-mental-health-interview/
3. Baliker M. Maria never gives up: are you brave like me? Scotts Valley: CreateSpace Independent Publishing Platform; 2017.

4. Beecher HK. The powerful placebo. JAMA J Am Med Assoc. 1955;159(17):1602–6. https://doi.org/10.1001/jama.1955.02960340022006.
5. Benedetti F, Mayberg HS, Wager TD, Stohler CS, Zubieta JK. Neurobiological mechanisms of the placebo effect. J Neurosci. 2005;25(45):10390–402. https://doi.org/10.1523/JNEUROSCI.3458-05.2005.
6. Boulay SD. Cicely Saunders: the founder of the modern hospice movement. London: SPCK Publishing; 2007.
7. Caan N. First African American full face transplant recipient advocates for organ donors and medical racial parity. 2024. https://www.plasticsurgery.org/news/articles/first-african-american-full-face-transplant-recipient-advocates-for-organ-donors-and-medical-racial-parity
8. Chida Y, Hamer M, Wardle J, Steptoe A. Do stress-related psychosocial factors contribute to cancer incidence and survival? Nat Clin Pract Oncol. 2008;5(8):466–75. https://doi.org/10.1038/ncponc1134.
9. Clark D. Cicely Saunders – founder of the hospice movement: selected letters 1959–1999. Oxford: Oxford University Press; 2002.
10. Cousins N. Anatomy of an illness as perceived by the patient: reflections on healing and regeneration. New York: Open Road Media; 2016.
11. Dickinson E. Poems: series two. Boston: Roberts Brothers; 1891.
12. Doctor comforting elderly patient in heartbreaking photo speaks out. CNN. 2020. Retrieved March 31, 2025 from https://www.cnn.com/videos/us/2020/11/30/elderly-patient-thanksgiving-coronavirus-intv-berman-newday-vpx.cnn
13. Fogarty LA, Curbow BA, Wingard JR, McDonnell K, Somerfield MR. Can 40 seconds of compassion reduce patient anxiety? J Clin Oncol. 1999;17(1):371–9. https://doi.org/10.1200/JCO.1999.17.1.371.
14. Frankl V. Man's search for meaning. Boston: Beacon Press; 2006.
15. Groopman J. The anatomy of hope: how people prevail in the face of illness. New York: Random House; 2003.
16. Hillenbrand L. Unbroken: a world war II story of survival, resilience, and redemption. New York: Random House; 2010.
17. Kalanithi P. When breath becomes air. New York: Random House; 2016.
18. Kaptchuk TJ, Friedlander E, Kelley JM, Sanchez MN, Kokkotou E, Singer JP, Kowalczykowski M, Miller FG, Kirsch I, Lembo AJ. Placebos without deception: a randomized controlled trial in irritable bowel syndrome. PLoS One. 2010;5(12):e15591. https://doi.org/10.1371/journal.pone.0015591.
19. Lance Armstrong SJ. It's not about the bike: my journey Back to life. New York: Putnam Adult; 2000.
20. Lansing A. Endurance: Shackleton's incredible voyage. New York: Basic Books; 2014.
21. Lee K. Roslyn Singleton, Charlotte woman whose cancer battle went viral, dies at age 39. 2022. https://www.wfae.org/charlotte-area/2022-11-16/charlotte-woman-whose-cancer-battle-went-viral-dies-husband-says
22. Livingston T. An autobiography. South Carolina: Legare Street Press; 2022.
23. Lown B. The lost art of healing: practicing compassion in medicine. New York: Ballantine Books; 1999.
24. Macmillan M. An odd kind of fame: stories of Phineas Gage. Bradford: Bradford Books; 2002.
25. Peabody FW. The care of the patient. JAMA. 1927;88:877–82.
26. Segerstrom SC, Miller GE. Psychological stress and the human immune system: a meta-analytic study of 30 years of inquiry. Psychol Bull. 2004;130(4):601–30. https://doi.org/10.1037/0033-2909.130.4.601.
27. Skloot R. The immortal life of Henrietta lacks. New York: Random House Audio; 2010.
28. Snyder CR. Hope theory: rainbows in the mind. Psychol Inq. 2002;13(4):249–75.
29. Snyder CR, Rand KL, King EA, Feldman DB, Woodward JT. "False" hope. J Clin Psychol. 2002;58(9):1003–22. https://doi.org/10.1002/jclp.10096.
30. Support Resources for Adolescents and Young Adults (AYAs). https://www.mskcc.org/cancer-care/patient-education/adolescent-and-young-adult-support-resources

31. Tournier P. The healing of persons. Manhattan: Harper & Row; 1965.
32. Trudeau Institute history. Retrieved February 27, 2025, from https://www.trudeauinstitute.org/history?utm_source=chatgpt.com
33. TV+, A. (2022). In A. Keshishian, Selena Gomez: my mind & me.
34. Van Horn JD, Irimia A, Torgerson CM, Chambers MC, Kikinis R, Toga AW. Mapping connectivity damage in the case of Phineas Gage. PLoS One. 2012;7(5):e37454. https://doi.org/10.1371/journal.pone.0037454.

# Index




F. Aziz, *The Healing Art of Connecting with Patients*,
https://doi.org/10.1007/978-3-032-03624-7

MIX
Papier aus verantwortungsvollen Quellen
Paper from responsible sources
FSC® C105338

If you have any concerns about our products,
you can contact us on
**ProductSafety@springernature.com**

In case Publisher is established outside the EU,
the EU authorized representative is:
**Springer Nature Customer Service Center GmbH**
**Europaplatz 3, 69115 Heidelberg, Germany**

Printed by Libri Plureos GmbH
in Hamburg, Germany